POVERTY AND HEALTH

Working with Families

CLARE BLACKBURN

OPEN UNIVERSITY PRESS
Milton Keynes · Philadelphia

Open University Press
Celtic Court
22 Ballmoor
Buckingham
MK18 1XW

and
1900 Frost Road, Suite 101
Bristol, PA 19007, US

First Published 1991
Reprinted 1992

British Library Cataloguing-in-Publication Data

Blackburn, Clare
    Poverty and health: Working with families.
    I. Title
    362.5083

    ISBN 0-335-09735-9
    ISBN 0-335-09734-0 (pbk)

Library of Congress Cataloging in Publication Data

Blackburn, Clare. 1957-
    Poverty and health:working with families/Clare Blackburn.
        p.   cm.
    Includes index.
    ISBN 0-335-09735-9 (hc) ISBN 0-335-09734-0 (pb)
    1. Poverty—Health aspects. 2. Poor—Health and hygiene.
    I. Title
    RA418.5.P6B53   1991
    362.1'08'6942–dc20   91-21914 CIP

Typeset by Rowland Phototypesetting Ltd, Bury St Edmunds, Suffolk
Printed in Great Britain by St Edmundsbury Press Ltd,
Bury St Edmunds, Suffolk

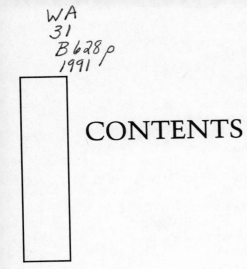

CONTENTS

ACKNOWLEDGEMENTS

I would like to thank a number of people whose support and help have enriched this book. Foremost, I would like to thank Hilary Graham whose support and guidance were invaluable. I also owe my thanks to members of the Health Promotion in Poverty Project Development and Evaluation Group who took the time to read and comment on drafts of the book: Dorit Braun, Jill Blackshaw, Kate Brown, Ann James, Mary Jones, Moira Keyes, Gwen Mellon, Heather Page, Kamlesh Sharman and Sylvie Summer. Ann Phoenix and Shantu Watt also gave valuable feedback that was much appreciated. Thanks also to Norma Baldwin and Ruth Elkan for all the encouragement and support they gave when the going got tough. Elizabeth Leed provided help with the preparation of the manuscript. A special thanks to Pete Hyde for help with the line drawings and your support. Finally, I am in debt to the Health Promotion Research Trust, who provide the funding for the Health Promotion in Poverty Project. The views expressed in this book are those of the author and not necessarily those of the Trust or those who provided guidance and support.

Figures 3.1 and 4.2 and tables 5.1 and 5.3 are reproduced with the permission of the Controller, HMSO and subject to Crown copyright.

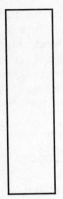

INTRODUCTION

This book is concerned with the impact of poverty on health. It focuses on one particular group in poverty: families with young children. It does so because the relationship between poverty and health is a particularly important issue with respect to families with young children. Poverty levels have risen sharply since 1979 amongst families with children. Families with dependent children now form the largest single group in poverty. At one of the most crucial life-stages, a substantial number of families have incomes and living conditions that are not compatible with good health.

The book seeks to bring together a rich seam of information and insights on poverty and the health of families with young children. A growing body of research has pointed to the way poverty affects the health chances and health choices of those who experience it. This literature has underlined the need for those who work with families to understand and respond more effectively to the health and welfare needs that family poverty creates. Whilst a rich source of material on poverty and family health exists, it has not been readily available to health and welfare workers. *Poverty and Health: Working with Families* attempts to bring together this material, and make it accessible to those who are concerned about the health of families with young children. The book draws together literature from within and across a wide range of disciplines – social policy, sociology, psychology, biological sciences, medicine, and health promotion – which can inform and guide health and welfare practice. It uses both 'hard' and 'soft' data in the acknowledgment that we need not only 'facts and figures' but first-hand accounts if we are to understand how poverty impacts on family health and family life.

Poverty and Health: Working with Families is concerned with the kinds of issues and questions that health and welfare workers confront on a daily basis in their work with families. It is written by someone who comes from health and welfare practice, for practitioners who face similar dilemmas, constraints and concerns in their work. It is written with the information needs of the multitude of family workers in mind, including social workers, health visitors, community nurses, school nurses, nursery workers, community workers and education workers. Drawing together the literature on poverty and health, the book is designed to be of interest to students on courses which include health and welfare studies.

This book seeks to provide workers with access to materials which will help them to deepen their understanding of the complex interconnections between living conditions, lifestyles and the health problems associated with poverty. In doing so, it draws out some of the issues for fieldwork practice and makes some suggestions concerning how health and welfare work can become more responsive to the needs of families in poverty. It does not, however, offer any blueprint for practice. The wealth of information available from research studies and the accounts of families make it clear that fieldwork strategies need to be worked out with individual communities and within and across agencies according to local need. Whilst families share some common experiences of poverty, their experiences differ according to a number of factors including family structure, gender, ethnic group, housing location, degree of social integration and level of social support. To offer a blueprint for practice would be to deny, first, the diversity of family life and family poverty and, second, to ignore the complex decisions that fieldworkers have to make, and the contradictions they face in their work.

The book seeks to address the central question 'Does poverty affect the health of those who experience it, and if so, how?' In order to answer this question it addresses a series of other questions along the way. Chapter 1 sets the scene for the rest of the book by examining the extent and causes of poverty in Britain today. This chapter begins by addressing the question 'What is poverty?' It does so in the recognition that the term poverty is a controversial term with several meanings. The sense in which the term is used is shaped by beliefs and current opinion about the nature of poverty. It is essential to explore the meaning of the term before moving on to assess the extent of poverty in Britain, and ask the questions 'Who are the poor?' and 'What makes people poor in a relatively prosperous industrial society?' This chapter explores how family structure, 'race' and gender influence a family's likelihood of being in poverty.

Chapter 2 moves on to ask the question 'What are the links between poverty and ill-health?' This chapter begins by examining the differences in health status between different groups in society – between social classes, between different ethnic groups and between men and women. It shows how those groups with the lowest incomes also have the poorest health. The chapter shows how household income is a key health resource for families. By focusing on the role of household income in health it is possible to begin to discover what it is about social class, gender, and 'race' that influences a person's health status. This chapter also introduces a framework within which the health effects of poverty can be analysed. It explores how poverty affects health through three interconnected processes – physiological, psychological and behavioural. In reality, these processes are not separate or clearly defined, and it is important to recognize that the book separates them out merely as a way of helping the reader to understand that the relationship between health and poverty is complex and cannot be explained by concentrating on any one dimension alone.

Chapters 1 and 2 are introductory chapters which set the scene for the rest of the book. The four chapters which follow examine the question 'How does poverty affect the health of those who experience it?' In doing so, they seek to draw out how the health effects of poverty stem from the fact that poor families do not have access to healthy living conditions: they do not have access to the financial and material resources that enable them to make healthy choices. These chapters explore specific health issues – nutrition and food, housing and health, mental health and caring for children's health – to illustrate the links between poverty and poor health. Finally, chapter 7 summarizes the main themes and evidence and draws out of the material some of the main issues for social policy and health and welfare practice.

Although the book draws together a wide range of material on poverty and family health, it does not aim – or claim – to be a definitive text on the subject. It is selective in the literature sources and issues it examines. It selects the research studies that help the reader to identify and understand a key set of issues in the poverty and health debate. In selecting some issues for detailed consideration the book, inevitably, excludes an in-depth discussion of others. It concentrates on the issues that most clearly demonstrate the complex interconnections between family poverty and poor health. It does so not because the issues it devotes less time to are any less important, but because the lessons we learn by exploring one dimension of poverty can often be applied to other dimensions of poverty. The book is also selective in the sense that it explores poverty and ill health by focusing on family access to household income. However, the author recognizes that other factors, such as level of education, also influence access to resources and life chances. The materials concentrate on the role of income in health because household income can be shown to be a key health resource that acts as a gatekeeper to other health resources, including housing, food, transport and heating. A focus on the role of income in health and illness is relatively unexplored in the research literature, particularly in comparison to the links between social position and health. Yet this focus has considerable explanatory power and offers us the opportunity to begin to unpack what it is about social position that influences health chances and deepens our understanding of why health inequalities persist and have widened in a relatively wealthy nation.

However, selectivity is not an excuse for omission. The blame for some omissions lies with the author: other omissions reflect the gaps in research on poverty and health. There are some clear gaps in the data sources that need to be attended to by the research community. For example, we need to know more about intra-household poverty, and, particularly, the distribution of resources within Black and minority ethnic families. Lack of available material in some areas has also meant that the book has sometimes had to move beyond the data in its search for ways of understanding family life. For example, in the chapter on stress, mental health and poverty, the material attempts to make some sense of a diverse range of research literature that is relevant to an exploration of poverty and health, but which does not always directly concern itself with it.

It is useful to note how various key terms are used in the text. The term 'family' is used to describe a group of individuals who live together and use the same household resources. Thus the term refers to a social grouping of people rather than a natural, or biological, grouping of people. It does so in the recognition that there are many different family structures and forms of family life and acknowledges that no one type or structure is necessarily any more legitimate than another.

The term 'Black' is used to refer to people of Afro-Caribbean and Asian descent. It is not used simply as an alternative to non-white, but to portray a common unity that is forged out of the experience of racism in British society. A capital B is used to indicate that the term Black refers to the social and political identity of being Black rather than the colour of people's skin. The materials use this term in the belief that it is one that is increasingly being used by many Black people themselves. Whilst this term is currently acceptable, its suitability may change over time. By using the term Black, the author does not wish to deny the diversity of cultures and ethnicities that together form Britain's Black population. Where appropriate in the literature ethnic groups are referred to separately.

The term 'minority ethnic' is used to refer to groups who are not necessarily Black, but who, like Black groups, are a minority in the numerical sense, and in the sense that they have minimal power in comparison to the majority ethnic group, for example, groups of Irish, Chinese and Polish origin. Again, there is a danger of denying the diversity of groups by using this term. Thus it should be borne in mind when reading this term that it refers to groups that each have their own cultural identity, history and way of life.

The word 'race' is written in inverted commas to signify that it is referring to social distinctions between groups rather than biological distinctions.

The term 'health' is used to refer to a broad concept, where health is about more than the absence of disease and illness and includes a sense of personal physical, mental and social well-being and the ability to reach one's potential.

The changing climate of unpaid and paid health work provides the background to this book. A growing number of families with young children have found it increasingly difficult to maintain a standard of living which is compatible with health. High unemployment and low pay levels have increased the number of households with young children with low household incomes. As some contributory parts of the benefits system have been weakened, for example, unemployment benefit, more people have become dependent on means-tested benefits. Benefits make an important contribution to the incomes of the poorest families, yet social-security benefits, the so-called safety net of the welfare state, remain set at very low levels. In many cases the evidence suggests that benefit levels are incompatible with good health.

Cuts in public expenditure have meant, in many areas, that there has been little investment in more public services, such as provision of council housing, childcare and transport, that are important to the health of Britain's poor families. Poor housing conditions, homelessness, unsafe housing locations, environmental dangers, inadequate transport systems and poor access to social and health services continue to be some of the problems that affect poor families disproportionately.

There have been changes, too, in the way professional work with families is structured. Social-service departments, local health services and voluntary agencies are experiencing more requests from families for help with financial and other material problems. Yet, while demands are increasing, changes to the social-security system have removed many of the mechanisms through which workers in the past were able to assist families to gain financial help, for example, through the single-payments system. Moreover, reforms emanating from the National Health Service and Community Care Act (1990) and the White Paper *Caring for People* (1989) have reshaped the roles and responsibilities of many family workers.

Together, the deteriorating material circumstances of families and new directions for health and welfare work have led to new challenges for those who work with families. The pressure for health and welfare workers to understand the links between poverty and health is greater than ever. Whilst the climate in which health and welfare workers currently operate offers little opportunity for radical change, it is important that workers maximize the opportunities they do have to support families in poverty and do not lose sight of what can be done when the social climate changes.

Note on the book
This book is free standing, but complements *Improving Health and Welfare Practice With Families in Poverty: A Handbook for Community Workers* by the same author which is to be published by Open University Press in the Spring of 1992. This second book contains a set of training materials that examine health and welfare strategies in relation to families in poverty.

1 | POVERTY: SETTING THE SCENE

INTRODUCTION

In the last decade poverty levels have dramatically risen in the United Kingdom, particularly among families with children. Poor families are the main users of social services and place high demands on health services, housing departments and voluntary organizations. But 'poverty' and 'the poor' are not neutral terms. They are highly controversial terms whose meanings are shaped by beliefs and current opinion about the nature and cause of poverty. Without doubt, there has been a revival of interest in the term 'poverty' in the last decade. As the effects of high levels of unemployment, low pay, regressive taxation policies, and changes to housing, health and social-security policies on families have become visible, poverty has once again found a place on the political agenda. Not only have poverty levels risen, but the climate in which families look after their health has changed. Cuts in public expenditure and extensive restructuring of the welfare state have rolled back the frontiers of the welfare state, placing responsibility for health and welfare firmly back with the family and individual. Self-help, family care and reliance on private and voluntary agencies are strong threads running through policies of the last decade.

Health and welfare workers are increasingly confronting complex and controversial issues relating to poverty.[1] Poverty and health are intrinsically linked. Not only are the poor more likely to suffer ill health and premature death, but poor health and disability are themselves recognized to be causes of poverty. Whilst there have been undeniable improvements in health in the post-war years, inequalities in health have widened, with the poor experiencing the fewest improvements in health. Although there is a growing acknowledgement that poverty is linked to health, much health and welfare practice fails to have any strategic impact on family poverty. The historical development of many health and welfare professions has resulted in practice based on finding individual solutions to the problems of poor health and poverty. Fieldwork responses are often fragmented, with each agency focusing on a separate set of presenting problems rather than on the problem of poverty itself. Moreover, the same policies that have reduced the resources for families to care have also made it increasingly difficult for health and welfare work to break out of models of intervention that concentrate on individual behaviour, and towards models that acknowledge the social and economic consequences of poverty for family life.

Health and welfare workers' beliefs about the nature and causes of poverty influence how they work at two levels. At the individual level, their beliefs influence what they do and how they treat clients. At the organizational level, social and political beliefs about poverty shape the boundaries and objectives of their agencies. Moreover, how poverty is conceptualized influences who is identified and counted as being 'poor'. The fact that poverty is an everyday reality for a growing number of families means that work with families needs to be based on a clear understanding of the meaning, causes and dimensions of poverty in Britain today.

This chapter aims to provide those who are concerned with the health of families with young children with a greater understanding of the issues surrounding poverty. To set the scene for the rest of the book, this chapter will cover the following areas:

- *Concepts of poverty*: discussing the different meanings that are associated with the term poverty, and the importance of seeing poverty as a relative concept.
- *Measuring poverty*: examining the problems inherent in measuring whom we identify and count as 'poor'.
- *Patterns of poverty in the United Kingdom today*: highlighting how poverty is not evenly distributed between different social groups.
- *The causes of relative poverty in the United Kingdom (UK)*.

WHAT IS POVERTY?

Before any assessment of the extent and dimensions of poverty in the UK can be made, it is important to clarify what we mean by the term 'poverty'. A number of different meanings have been given to the term, and there has been considerable controversy about which is the most acceptable way to define it.

There appear to be two broad ways of viewing poverty – as an absolute concept, and as a relative concept. These concepts are based on different ways of seeing people's needs[2] and affect views about what resources should be allocated to the poor. Page 9 gives some key definitions of poverty.

Some key definitions of poverty

Families are in poverty when their incomes are 'insufficient to obtain the minimum necessities for the maintenance of physical efficiency'.

B. S. Rowntree, 1941[3]

Individuals, families, and groups can be said to be in poverty when they lack the resources to obtain the types of diet, participate in the activities and have the living conditions and amenities which are customary, or at least widely encouraged or approved, in the societies to which they belong.

P. Townsend, 1979[4]

Persons are beset by poverty when 'resources are so small as to exclude them from the minimum acceptable way of life of the Member State in which they live'.

Council of Ministers, EEC, 1981[5]

. . . A family is in poverty if it cannot afford to eat.

K. Joseph and J. Sumption, 1979[6]

ABSOLUTE POVERTY

The concept of absolute poverty, sometimes known as primary poverty, was developed in the late nineteenth century when government and ruling groups felt under pressure to define the minimum needs of the poor in and outside poor-law institutions. This concept is closely associated with the work of the social reformer Seebohm Rowntree.

The concept of absolute poverty rests on the idea that it is possible to define a minimum standard for physical survival, and that the needs of the poor do not change through time. These ideas were adopted in William Beveridge's plans for the post-war social-security system (against Rowntree's advice) and formed the basis of national assistance (later supplementary benefit and now income support). The national assistance scheme was designed to keep those dependent on it out of poverty and appears to have been set at a minimum level of subsistence.

The concept of absolute poverty remains a powerful one in the UK today and is thought by many social scientists to be the basis for the social-security system. The concept still has many supporters (although few in academic circles) and is often used to argue that there is no real poverty in Britain today. In a speech entitled 'The end of the line for poverty' (May, 1989) John Moore, Social Security Secretary, said poverty in the 'old and absolute sense of hunger and want' had been wiped out. He suggests that, if poverty, as defined by the Victorian social reformers, does not exist, then it is no longer useful to speak of it.[7]

Critics of this view object to the assertion that poverty should be defined narrowly in terms of nineteenth-century Britain. Poverty is not only about what you need to avoid dying from starvation and cold, but the conditions you need to stay healthy and participate in the society in which you need to live. Although the concept of absolute poverty has applicability in parts of the Developing World, where famine is an overriding concern, an alternative concept is needed to assess poverty in the Western world in the 1990s:

> Poor people in Britain are not, of course, as poor as those in the Third World, but their poverty is real enough nonetheless. For poverty is a relative as well as an absolute concept. It exists even in a relatively rich western society, if people are denied access to what is generally regarded as a reasonable standard and quality of life in Society.[8]

RELATIVE POVERTY

The idea that poverty is relative to the kind of society we live in at a particular time has been developed at length by Townsend as an alternative to the view that poverty can be assessed in terms of the customs and standards of a previous era, or seen in absolute terms. Absolute rises in income are not enough if families are still unable to afford resources for good health. Townsend suggested that people are in poverty when they:

> lack the resources to obtain the type of diet, participate in the activities, and have the living conditions and amenities which are customary, or at least widely encouraged or approved in the society in which they belong.[9]

This implies that poverty is about being poor in comparison to the standard of living of others, and about being unable to do the things that are generally accepted as part of a way of life:

> Now he is at school, and tells me about other children's bikes, and the toys they take, and holidays, and days out with parents, and it breaks my heart for there is nothing for him; if he has food and clothes he can have nothing else.
>
> (A single parent with a 5-year-old son)[10]

Here, poverty is concerned with social needs as well as physical needs. People are social beings, with social roles and relationships. Our needs arise through these roles and relationships, as well as through our need for physical survival. Personal accounts suggest that poverty hinders people in their roles and relationships: as parents, friends, partners, active citizens, or supportive neighbours. Household income not only determines access to amenities, lifestyles, and choices, it also regulates access to power structures. Families on low household income often find it difficult to afford the transport and other costs of attending local-authority council meetings, school meetings or pressure groups meeting; thus they lose the opportunity to challenge decisions and policies that affect them. Like health, poverty is a wider concept than the absence of physical symptoms.

The idea that poverty is relative to today's standards, and about more than physical needs, appears to be a view shared outside as well as inside academic circles. A MORI poll conducted for London Weekend Television in 1983 found that, first, large numbers of the population in Britain make decisions about what constitutes a minimum standard of living on social criteria (for example, having enough money to buy birthday presents), and not just on criteria for physical survival. Second, it highlighted that there is a public consensus that necessities for living are judged on today's standards and not those of the past:[11]

9 out of 10 people saw the following as necessities:
- heating
- indoor toilet (not shared)
- damp-free home
- a bath (not shared)
- beds for everyone

2 out of 3 people saw the following as necessities:
- enough money for public transport
- 3 meals a day for children
- 2 pairs of all-weather shoes and a warm winter coat
- a refrigerator and washing machine
- enough money for special occasions (e.g. Christmas and birthdays)

Here we can see how financial poverty is associated with, and compounded by, poor access to other resources. Income is a key resource for families. It determines access to a host of other resources for health. Families with low incomes are least able to afford, or have access to, good housing conditions. They have little choice about the type of accommodation they live in, or where they live. Families in poverty are more likely to be living in rented accommodation that is insecure, overcrowded and in poor structural condition than higher-income families. Moreover, poor families are likely to live in less hospitable areas, with poor access to safe play areas, and health, education and leisure services. Poverty-level incomes do not enable families to buy the foods that are thought to be important for health, or pay for enough heating to keep homes warm and free from damp and condensation. Families in poverty cannot afford family outings or goods that make life more bearable and are important for mental and physical health. Families on low incomes can often afford only poor-quality equipment and furnishings that are badly designed, wear out or break quickly. For families using credit facilities, goods may wear out or break even before they are paid for. Cheap goods not only lack the quality of more expensive goods, but also frequently fail to meet the same safety standards.

Above all, poverty is an experience – an experience of 'doing without' – that touches every part of life and family health care. These dimensions of poverty, and the way they impact on the health of families, will be discussed in future chapters.

Although the concepts of absolute poverty and relative poverty are based on different ways of seeing people's needs, they share an approach that defines and measures poverty at the level of the household unit. The concept of poverty we operate with is important, not only in the sense that it affects how we view the needs of the poor, but also because it influences how we measure the amount of poverty that exists in society.

MEASURING POVERTY

Being in poverty means not having a level of income to sustain health, and being out of poverty means having a level of income which is compatible with health.[12] The most common way to measure poverty is in terms of household income, as income determines access to the amenities and resources that are important for good health. There is no official poverty line in the UK. However, if we wish to differentiate those who are poor from their better-off counterparts, it is necessary to draw a line between the two. Where we draw the line depends on how we define poverty and what we view as a minimum level of income and standard of living for families and individuals.

SLIPPERY STATISTICS

Two unofficial poverty lines help to measure the level of poverty in society and identify those with poverty level incomes. *The most extensively used poverty line uses the level of supplementary benefit (SB) as a bench-mark of poverty.* (Although this benefit no longer exists, the latest figures available relate to the period when supplementary benefit was available. Future statistics are likely to use the income-support level as the poverty line.) Although the level of benefits is, in many ways, an arbitrary figure, it represents a political decision about the distribution of wealth and, by implication, health, in our society. It can be argued that this figure represents a minimum level of income below which society believes incomes should not fall.

A wealth of evidence suggests that the levels of supplementary benefit/ income support have been set too low to maintain family health. Research indicates that 140 per cent of supplementary benefit/income support is a more adequate measure of poverty and represents the cut-off point between 'poverty' and 'welfare'.[13,14] Thus British studies traditionally define poverty in the following terms:

Anyone with an income on or below the level of supplementary benefit/income support (100 per cent of benefit level) is defined as living 'in poverty'.

Anyone with an income between 100–140 per cent of supplementary benefit/income support is defined as living 'on the margins of poverty'.

Figures for the numbers of individuals and households with incomes below 100 per cent and 140 per cent of supplementary benefit used to be available from a set of official statistics called the *Low Income Family Statistics*. These were published until 1988 (latest figures relate to 1985) by the Department of Health and Social Security.[15] Although the government used the bench-mark of 100–140 per cent of supplementary-benefit level as the bench-mark for low income, rather than poverty, these statistics were frequently used as measures of poverty by anti-poverty groups and voluntary and statutory bodies. Poverty statistics are also often used as a way of measuring the performance of a government. It is hardly surprising therefore that poverty statistics are politically sensitive and the subject of much controversy. As poverty levels began to rise substantially in the 1980s, the government became increasingly sensitive over the use of the *Low Income Family Statistics*. They argued that they were not an accurate measure of low income levels as, every time they increased the rate of supplementary benefit in real terms, that is, above the rate of inflation, the number of people defined as having a low income automatically increased as more people found themselves with incomes on or below 140 per cent of the new supplementary-benefit rate. The government decided not to publish the *Low Income Family Statistics* after 1988, despite protests from anti-poverty groups and the Social Services Select Committee who have both argued that this set of statistics are valuable and should be continued. However, the Institute for Fiscal Studies,[16] an independent organization, has subsequently published a broadly similar set of statistics based on the supplementary-benefit levels. The government has replaced the *Low Income Family Statistics* with a set of statistics called *Households Below Average Income Statistics*.

The *Households Below Average Income Statistics* use a new set of goal posts to measure low income. They show how the incomes of people in the lower half of the income distribution relate to average incomes. A measure, based on *Households Below Average Income Statistics*, is now being used by anti-poverty groups as a second poverty line. This measure uses 50 per cent of average income as the poverty line:

Anyone with an income on or below 50 per cent of average income is defined as living 'in poverty'.

Anyone with an income between 50–60 per cent of average income is defined as 'on the margins of poverty'.

There are advantages and disadvantages to using both poverty lines. Using the level of supplementary benefit/income support as a poverty line is useful because it uses the benefit-assessment unit (the family) as the unit of measure. This is generally thought to be more appropriate than using the household as the unit of measure (as used in the *Households Below Average Income Statistics*), as more than one family unit, with different income levels may live in a household. Using the level of supplementary benefit/income support also allows us to measure how many people have incomes below a minimum level that is set by government. However, a drawback is that any poverty statistics using this measure after 1988 are not based on an official set of government statistics and thus are less likely to be acceptable to government.

The second poverty line – below 50 per cent of average income – has an advantage in that it can be calculated from an official set of government figures. Moreover, it is a poverty line that is used by the European Community; thus European comparisons are now easier. However, this second measure has the drawback that it uses household income, as opposed to family income, as the unit of measure. The Institute for Fiscal Studies has calculated that, by using this unit, the figures grossly underestimate the numbers of people living on or below 50–60 per cent of average income.[17] Furthermore, using this poverty line means that, if average incomes fall, the figures would show a fall in the number of people in poverty, even though those in poverty may be worse off in real terms. Both poverty lines can be criticized because they are based on levels of income that are unacceptably low. The level of benefit and 50 per cent of average income are both very low levels of income. As we shall see in later chapters, they do not allow families to have access to the level of resources that they need for their health. Furthermore, both poverty lines do not address such questions as the distribution of poverty between different ethnic groups, between men and women or between members of the same family or household. Nor do they give us any information about the numbers of poor people who are homeless. As we shall see in this chapter, poverty levels differ significantly between these groups.

PATTERNS OF POVERTY

As there is no one straightforward way to measure poverty, this section will use both poverty lines to show current poverty levels and the distribution of poverty between different groups. *The figures show us that, regardless of which poverty line we use, there has been a substantial rise in the number of people in poverty since 1979.* From 1979 to 1987 the percentage of the population with incomes on or below a 140 per cent of supplementary benefit increased from 22 per cent to 28 per cent. In the same period, the percentage of people with incomes on or below 60 per cent of average

FIGURE 1.1   Numbers (thousands) and percentages of people living on or below margins of poverty in Britain, 1979 and 1987

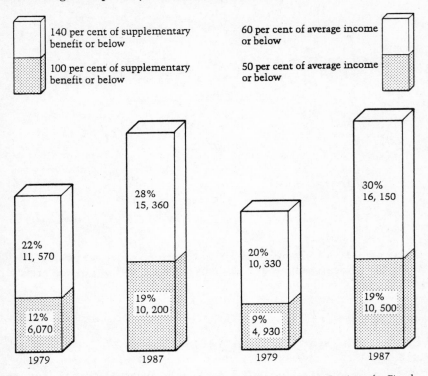

140 per cent of supplementary benefit or below

100 per cent of supplementary benefit or below

60 per cent of average income or below

50 per cent of average income or below

1979   1987   1979   1987

Sources: Johnson, P. and Webb, S. (1990). Poverty in Official Statistics. Institute for Fiscal Studies Commentary no. 24. London, Institute for Fiscal Studies.
Department of Social Security (1990). Households Below Average Income Statistics. London, HMSO.

income increased from 20 per cent to 30 per cent of the population (see figure 1.1).

The figures indicate different levels of poverty because they are measuring different things. The measure of 100–140 per cent of supplementary benefit indicates that, since 1979, more people have an income that falls below a minimum level. Although a slight rise in the value of supplementary benefit in this period accounts for some of this increase, it cannot explain it all. The Institute for Fiscal Studies[18] suggest that two-thirds of this increase are due to a rise in the number of people who are unemployed. By using the measure, 50 per cent of average earnings, we can see that more people have incomes that fall below the average income in 1987 than in 1979. Although average incomes have risen sharply in this period, the poorest groups have not benefited as much as better-off groups. Whilst

FIGURE 1.2   Proportion of people living in poverty (using 50 per cent of average income as the poverty line) by family type, 1987

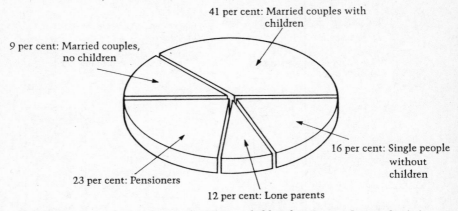

Source: Department of Social Security (1990) Households Below Average Income Statistics. London, HMSO.

average incomes have risen by 23 per cent, the incomes of the poorest 10 per cent of the population have only risen by 0.1 per cent (both figures are after housing costs).[19]

WHO ARE THE POOR?

Poverty is not evenly distributed between groups. The way society is organized and the effects of social policies render certain groups of people vulnerable to poverty. *The data tells us that unemployed and low-paid people, sick people, people with disabilities, older adults and families with children made up the main groups living in poverty in the UK in 1987.*

A significant feature of the 1980s is the fact that there has been a redistribution of poverty among those groups of people most vulnerable to it. The burden of poverty has shifted away from older people on to families with young children. Figure 1.2 shows the distribution of poverty by family type in 1987. Although the numbers of older people in poverty has remained much the same since 1979, they now form a smaller proportion of people living in, or on, the margins of poverty. There are several reasons for this. First, state pensions have fared slightly better than other state benefits in recent years; and in addition, a growing number of older people have occupational pensions to supplement their state pension. Second, high unemployment has dramatically increased the number of people of non-pensionable age in poverty, a growing number of whom live in families with dependent children and rely on state benefits, set at subsistence levels, as their main source of income.

The figures also tell us that the number of children living in families with incomes on or below the margins of poverty has increased significantly. At a crucial time in their lives a substantial number of children are living in or on the margins of poverty:

From 1979 to 1987 the percentage of children living in families on or below 140 per cent of supplementary benefit level increased from 18 per cent (2,370,000) to 30 per cent (3,610,000) of all children in 1987.

From 1979 to 1987 the proportion of children living in families with incomes below 50 per cent of average income increased from 12 per cent (1,620,000) to 26 per cent (3,090,000) in 1987.

To understand the changing pattern of poverty in Britain, we need to look at the effect that family structure, and the divisions of gender and 'race' have on family income and the distribution of resources between family members.

FAMILY STRUCTURE, GENDER AND 'RACE'

A growing proportion of the poor can be found among families headed by lone parents. One-parent families appear to be more likely than two-parent families to be in poverty. Although the proportion of lone-parent families is still relatively small (14 per cent of all families with dependent children), the proportion is growing rapidly. Since 1961 the number has doubled as there has been an increase in the number of births to single mothers and a rising divorce rate.[20] Changing marriage and divorce patterns mean that parents and children are likely to move in and out of one-parent families over a period of time. Although only a small minority of children live in one-parent families at any one time, many more will experience life in a lone-parent family during their childhood and adolescent years. By implication, this means that a growing proportion of children will spend part of their formative years living in, or on the margins of, poverty.

In 1987, 70 per cent of children in one-parent families compared to 13 per cent of children in two-parent families were living in, or on the margins of, poverty (using 100–140 per cent of SB as measure).

The average total weekly income for a lone-parent family in 1986 was less than half (40 per cent) of that of a comparable two-parent family, yet the major expenses of housing, food and costs relating to children were likely to be the same.[21]

The influence of family structure on income is compounded by gender and 'race' inequalities. The high proportion of one-parent families dependent on means-tested benefits is primarily due to the fact that the majority of lone parents (90 per cent) are women. Women's poorer access to the labour market and well-paid jobs, coupled with childcare costs, means that many lone mothers (53 per cent) are forced to rely on means-tested benefits. In general, lone fathers are more able than lone mothers to continue to earn a reasonable income after separation, due to their higher status and higher pay in the labour market. Lone mothers from Black and minority ethnic groups share many of the economic and social penalties of lone motherhood with white lone mothers but face the additional penalties that stem from the daily experience of racism. Personal and institutional racism appears to reduce the income of Black and minority ethnic women even further, increasing their propensity towards poverty. The tendency to treat Black families as pathological (particularly families with Black lone mothers) still persists and needs to be seen as a further factor that oppresses Black women and their children.

The differences in income between one- and two-parent families have been much more clearly documented than the differences within families. *Statistics ignore the fact that poverty can occur within families whose income brings them above the poverty line.* This phenomenon is often referred to as hidden poverty. The victims of hidden poverty are usually women.[22] Poverty is not a gender-neutral term. Research has shown that, even in high-income families, women can be poor within marriage regardless of their male partners' income.[23]

> Personally, I feel better off. Although we've got a lot less money in the family I feel better off because I can control it, you know. When I was married he used to give me so much a week and if I wanted anything else, I had to go and ask him and then say what it was, where it was, and how much it cost and then he may say, 'No, you can't have it'! So I feel a lot better off.
>
> (A separated mother with two children, living on supplementary benefit)[24]

In and out of marriage, women's household and family responsibilities, and their position in the economy, make them particularly vulnerable to poverty. Some authors suggest that this is a recent phenomenon – a 'feminization' of poverty where the burden of poverty has shifted from men to women.[25] Other authors suggest that female poverty has been a constant fact, and that women's poverty, previously invisible, is now becoming more clearly seen.[26] Women not only experience more poverty than men but also face the tasks of managing scarce resources within the family, and protecting other family members from poverty's worst elements (see chapters 3, 4, 5 and 6). Women's poverty and their primary responsibility for caring makes them especially vulnerable to ill health.

Whilst women's poverty has been fairly well documented, far less attention has been paid to the relationship between 'race' and poverty. The paucity of information on the effect of 'race' on family income is notable and symbolic of research's failure to acknowledge 'race' as an important dimension of inequality.

Black and minority ethnic groups have a greater-than-average likelihood of being on low income. Employment discrimination reduces access to employment and well-paid jobs, forcing a high proportion of ethnic-minority families to rely on social-security benefits set at subsistence levels. Many people from Black and minority ethnic groups report difficulties in claiming social-security benefits. A number of surveys have shown that underclaiming of benefits is higher among Black people than white people. Racist assumptions operate in the benefit system. Access to social-security benefits and other material resources is dependent on the attitudes and values of social-security staff. Racist attitudes affect both the availability of information about entitlements, and decisions about the allocation of entitlements. Lack of information about the social-security system and the complexities of the system itself have been shown to be the main set of barriers to Black and minority ethnic groups.[27] Assumptions about the needs and resources of Black and minority ethnic families act as further barriers to claimants. It is still wrongly assumed that Black and minority ethnic groups are responsible for their own poverty. Social-security decisions also appear to be based on misconceptions about the organization of family and community networks. For example, claims have been invalidated because social-security staff have assumed that among Asian groups other family or community members can provide financial help. Racist assumptions also affect the access and allocation of other resources. For Black and minority ethnic groups poverty is often compounded by poor housing, poor health care and inner-city residence, as well as the personal experience of living in a climate of hostility.

CAUSES OF POVERTY

It is clear that, despite several years of economic growth, poverty is on the increase among families with young children. The 1980s were a decade of poverty amidst plenty. A key question for health and welfare workers, politicians, and policy-makers alike is 'What creates poverty in a relatively prosperous industrial society?' How we answer this question depends on our beliefs about the nature of poverty. The answer, in turn, affects the emphasis that policy-makers and politicians place on tackling poverty, and how health and welfare workers respond to the needs of their clients.

Dominant explanations in the past have regarded poverty as a consequence of the moral weakness or the psychological or social inadequacy of individuals.[28] Moralistic overtones are still present, encapsulated in the image of the 'welfare scrounger' and the attitude that the welfare state removes the incentive for people to help themselves. However, there is evidence to suggest that both public opinion,[29] and the opinion of some welfare workers[30] are inclined to identify social and economic factors as the cause of poverty. An ever-increasing amount of research and literature clearly identifies poverty with social and economic causes.

The way society is organized and the effect of social and economic policies influence the conditions under which people live and work and the amount of support available to enable people to meet their health and social needs. Family responsibilities, lone parenthood, old age and disability create extra needs: additional heating, suitable and easily accessible forms of transport, enough money for suitable clothing, safe and appropriate housing. The following four sub-sections will examine how high levels of unemployment, low pay, disability and taxation policies reduce the ability of many families with dependent children to meet their financial and material needs. The failure of the social-security benefits system to act as an adequate safety net at times of unemployment, low pay and disability will be discussed within these sub-sections.

UNEMPLOYMENT

Unemployment is still a major cause of poverty today. The real recent collapse of employment occurred in the early 1980s, when the effects of a world recession and a Conservative government's economic policies hit the job market.[31] There has been a fall in the official unemployment count since 1986, and the unemployment figure for May 1990 was 1.6 million.[32] It is suggested that the extent of the problem has been obscured: first, by the way government has changed the method of counting the unemployed; and second, by the fact that the unemployment figures do not take account of the number of people who are on government employment and training schemes.[33] The unemployment figures are another example of 'slippery statistics'.

> The government has changed its method of counting the unemployed 24 times in the nine years between 1979 and 1988. The aggregate effect has reduced the figures significantly.[34]

> New benefit regulations reduced the count by 90,000 in April 1988, when under-18-year-olds were no longer eligible for income support.

The burden of unemployment is not equally shared out among the population. Certain areas of the country and groups of individuals bear the brunt of the problem. A north–south divide remains, with the north of the country, Scotland and Northern Ireland having a considerably higher unemployment rate than the south. Some occupations have been affected more than others. Manual jobs in manufacturing industry and parts of the service sector have been particularly affected. Individuals with characteristics perceived as 'attractive' by employers (young, white, experienced workers with good health and qualifications) are likely to have the least risk of unemployment.[35]

The risk of unemployment is also related to gender. Women's unemployment has increased faster than male unemployment in the decade. Whereas male unemployment began to level off after 1983, women's unemployment continued to rise until 1986.

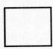 In February 1989, women's unemployment remained higher than men's at 9.1 per cent of the female population, compared to 7.1 per cent for men (seasonally unadjusted figures).[36]

Divisions of labour operate within paid employment. Women, unlike men, are not found across the spectrum of employment. Women are concentrated in a much narrower band of occupations than men. Women tend to be concentrated in jobs in caring and servicing, particularly jobs in the cleaning, clothing, hospital and clerical sectors. Women's employment tends to be different from men's employment in that it tends to be low paid, insecure and part-time. Cuts in public expenditure have had a significant effect on women's employment levels. The public-service sector (for example, the National Health Service, social-services departments, education services) is a large employer of women. First, spending cuts in these areas have reduced the number of jobs available to women. Second, cuts have reduced the numbers of day-nursery places; reduced pre-school provision; and increased the need for the sick, physically and mentally disabled, and old to be cared for at home. The result is to reduce women's opportunities to take up paid employment even further, as well as to increase the amount of unpaid domestic work for women.[37]

The risk of unemployment is also related to 'race'. Unemployment levels are higher among Black people. For example, people of West Indian origin have an unemployment rate twice that of the white population, while people of Pakistani and Bangladeshi origin have an unemployment rate three times as high. In addition, the more qualifications Black workers have appears to increase their relative disadvantage in the labour market. For example, highly qualified Pakistani and Bangladeshi men have an unemployment rate four times that of similarly qualified white workers.[38] Individual and institutional racism reduces the employment prospects of Black people, regardless of their qualifications and level of skill.

Black women face the dual oppression of sexism and racism in the labour market. They experience a different position in the labour market to both white women and men of all races.[39] Black women tend to be in jobs with the lowest pay and the poorest conditions. Phizacklea has suggested that Black women, who form a reserve army of labour, are both made redundant quickly during a recession and re-employed faster when the economy improves.[40] Black women tend to have high levels of participation in the labour market. This is thought to be related, in part, to the low wages of Black men. Homeworking is particularly common among women from Black and minority ethnic groups, particularly women from Asian groups. These jobs tend to be the lowest paid, least secure of all jobs, but allow women who face the greatest discrimination in the labour market and the poorest access to childcare resources to earn a wage that helps to raise the poverty-level incomes of their partners.

The unemployment figures reflect a picture of a particular moment in time. However, the unemployed are not a static mass of people. People move in and out of employment continuously. As a result, unemployment affects more families than the statistics suggest. A large number of people will experience a period of unemployment, and therefore poverty, at some time in their lives. Berthoud's study highlighted that there is no poorer group of people than unemployed couples with children, with the exception of the down-and-out homeless.[41] The unemployed are heavily dependent on income support. Having children incurs extra costs, yet income support rates remain too low to meet the costs of a child. The Child Poverty Action Group has calculated and published the minimum direct costs of providing children with food, clothing and other bare necessities and compared these costs with the personal allowances made to children through the income-support scheme.[42] For children of all ages the income-support allowances for children fall short of the estimated minimum costs of children.

Child benefit, the only non-means-tested payment made to families, has been shown to be an important source of additional income to mothers.[43] Yet, in 1990 it was frozen at 1987 rates for the third year running. Long-term unemployed families experience the worst poverty because clothes and household goods eventually need to be replaced. People classified as long-term unemployed no longer receive a higher rate of benefit, and the discontinuation of single payments to benefit claimants makes it particularly difficult to meet everyday living costs.

Since the introduction of the new income-support scheme in April 1988, claimants of income support have to cover costs which were previously met by the old supplementary-benefit scheme. These new costs include 20 per cent of water rates, household maintenance and insurance, and part of the poll tax. In addition, income-support claimants are no longer entitled to claim grants from the Department of Social Security (DSS) for essential items such as a bed or a cooker. The non-repayable single-payment scheme has been replaced by a money loan scheme. Loans are repayable through weekly deductions from benefit of between 15–25 per cent of the cost of the loan. There is no automatic right to a loan, with loan decisions depending on how a local social-fund manager views the merits of a case, and how much money is available at the time in the cash-limited social fund. Debt problems are likely to increase as more unemployed families are forced to use credit or borrow to cope with daily money-management problems.

LOW PAY

Low pay is now the biggest single cause of poverty in Britain today.[44] Like the definition of poverty, the definition of low pay is controversial and influences who is identified as 'low paid'. There are several definitions of low pay, all of which rest on the idea of a 'decency threshold', below which wages are classified as low pay. Some of these definitions, for instance the Low Pay Unit's definition, are based on relative levels of earnings, while others are based on absolute levels, such as family credit.

Many people move between unemployment and low-paid jobs. Whatever has happened to unemployment in the past decade, the problems of low pay continue to increase.

> Since 1979, the number of low-paid adult workers has increased from 38 per cent to around 48 per cent of the workforce.[45]

If the Low Pay Unit's definition of low pay as two-thirds of the median male wage or below an hourly rate of £3.80 (1989 figure) is used, approximately 9 million workers are low paid (see table 1.1).

The majority of Britain's low paid are women who make up two-thirds of the low paid. Women are less likely to be in well-paid jobs than men. They are also more likely to be in less secure part-time jobs, which fit in with their domestic and child care responsibility within the home. Four out of five women working part-time earn low wages. Unlike men, many women are unable to boost their pay by working overtime. Furthermore, women earn lower wages than men (around three-quarters of men's wages), whether they are in part-time or full-time jobs. Women's concentration in low-paid work results in particular hardship for lone mothers and families that rely on the woman to boost the family income. Women's low wages help to cushion their families from the impact of male low pay and have the effect of keeping many families out of poverty.[46]

A gap in the official statistics is an absence of any data on the earnings of different ethnic groups. However, evidence from a survey by the Policy Studies Institute suggests that Asian and West Indian men earned wages 15 per cent lower than white men.[47]

The social-security benefit, family credit, which replaced family income supplement in April 1988, is a means-tested benefit to help families on low income. Although many families may be entitled to this benefit, take up is very low. In September 1987 only a third of those thought to be entitled to family credit were receiving it.[48] Those that do claim it may find themselves

TABLE 1.1   Numbers and proportions of low-paid workers

How many people are low paid?

- 5 million full-time workers
- 4 million part-time workers
- 80 per cent of all part-time workers
- 66 per cent of all women workers

Source: Winyard, S. and Pond, C. (1989). *Ten Years On: The Poor Decade.* London, Low Pay Unit

in the 'poverty trap', where any rise in earnings results in lower income due to withdrawal of part or all of benefit payments, or an increase in taxation. Lone mothers in part-time and low-paid work are most likely to find themselves in this situation.

> As a single parent I don't earn enough to manage. As a nurse I'm poorly paid anyway. I'm in this poverty trap – if I earn over a certain amount I'm not entitled to any benefits.
>
>   (A single mother of two children)[49]

DISABILITY

Families of people with disabilities suffer a disproportionate risk of poverty. Disability and low income are closely linked. Disability creates extra needs: the need for extra heating, special food, transport, special aids, equipment and additional clothing. These extra needs incur costs which are above the costs incurred by families which have no people with disabilities:

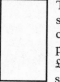

> The first Office of Population Censuses and Surveys (OPCS) survey of disability in Britain found that families with disabled children incurred regular additional average expenditures of £4.55 per week in the case of children with low disability scores and £12.53 per week for families with children with high disability scores.[50]

Yet many families of people with disabilities do not have incomes to cover these extra costs adequately. The 1988 OPCS survey of disability highlighted that families with people with disabilities have lower incomes than other equivalent families. For example, families containing adults of working age with disabilities had incomes that were only 72 per cent of the incomes of other equivalent families. Moreover, 34 per cent of families with adults of working age with disabilities had incomes below half the average income for the general population, compared to 23 per cent of equivalent non-disabled families.[51]

Income from employment is often restricted for adults with disabilities and members of their families. Many adults are prevented from working because of limited job opportunities for people with disabilities or because of the severity of their disability. Those who are employed are often in low-paid jobs or have low incomes because they work restricted hours due to their disability. Many relatives of people with disabilities, particularly women, also suffer loss of earnings. Caring for a child or adult with disabilities may make it difficult to go out to work. Relatives who are able to work may suffer loss of earnings due to the need to restrict working hours in order to carry out caring activities. Career moves that entail extra work, working away from home or job mobility may also be restricted.

Reduced access to income through employment, the absence of a comprehensive disability income and the inadequacy of benefits such as the invalidity benefit and attendance allowance means that many families with people with disabilities have to rely on means-tested social-security benefits. Yet means-tested benefits have received the harshest cuts in recent years. As a result of changes to supplementary benefit, housing benefit, and family income supplement, 80,000 sick and disabled people under pensionable age are worse off.[52] Families of children with disabilities in particular lose out under the new income-support scheme. The disabled child's premium is very small (£6.15 per week in 1989) and can be claimed only if the child is in receipt of attendance or mobility allowance or is registered blind. As some children are under the age limit for attendance or mobility allowance, they do not qualify for this premium, regardless of the severity of their disability. Until social-security benefits are based on need, rather than type of disability, age or place of occurrence, and until a comprehensive disability-income scheme exists, many families of people with disabilities will continue to live in or on the margins of poverty or have incomes that are significantly below those of equivalent other families.

TAXATION

The amount of taxation levied by government on individuals affects the amount of available income they have to spend on family health. Changes to direct taxation (income tax and national insurance contributions) between 1979 and 1988 have had the net effect of increasing the proportion of earnings taken in tax from the low paid. Hill's analysis of the combined effect of changes to direct taxation and benefits since the tax year 1978–9 indicates that the bottom 60 per cent of the income distribution have a weekly net loss, while the top 30 per cent have gained.[53] Indirect taxation (VAT, taxes on alcohol, tobacco and petrol) may also affect the poor disproportionately, although there has been little research in this area.

CONCLUSION AND IMPLICATIONS FOR PRACTICE

Three key points emerge from this chapter. First, it is important that those concerned with the health and welfare of families see poverty as a relative concept. As a relative concept, poverty becomes an issue that concerns more than minimum physical needs. It informs us that poverty creates social and emotional needs, relative powerlessness, and lack of freedom. Second, the research evidence and government statistics indicate that poverty is on the increase, particularly among families with young children. At the most crucial period in family life, an increasing number of parents and children are experiencing living conditions and levels of financial hardship that are not compatible with good health. Third, poverty stems from the way society is organized, and the effect of social and economic policies. Individual behaviour or characteristics cannot account for rising poverty levels. Social and economic policies do not affect all individuals and families equally. Some groups appear to benefit from these policies, whilst others, notably low-income groups, women of all ethnic groups, Black and minority ethnic groups of both sexes, and people with disabilities become further disadvantaged. Last, the causes of poverty indicate that the solutions to poverty are social and economic. The solutions involve not only increases in income for vulnerable groups, but a fundamental redistribution of wealth in society.

This chapter has documented the growing problem of poverty in Britain. Whilst poverty is once again a political 'hot potato', policies to reduce the level of poverty have failed to appear on the government's agenda during the last decade. The impact of poverty on families indicates that health and welfare workers cannot ignore the consequences of poverty for their clients, or the links between fieldwork practice and social and economic policies.

The structural nature of poverty may leave many health and welfare workers feeling helpless, or feeling that tackling poverty is beyond their remit. But poverty must be a central concern for fieldworkers. A substantial and growing area of health and welfare work is a reactive response to the impact of poverty on family life. Policies and interventions to reduce poverty are important in their own right – all families have an equal right to a level of financial and material resources to sustain family life. But poverty also has health costs – it affects the health and well-being of those who experience it. The following chapter will examine the current evidence on the relationship between poverty and health. It will place this evidence within a framework that will help those who work with families to develop their understanding of how poverty undermines health. It will show the scope there is for health and welfare work to help families fight the causes of poverty and avoid its worst effects.

REFERENCES

1 Becker, S. and MacPherson, S. (1988). *Public Issues, Private Pain.* London, Insight.
2 Oppenheim, C. (1988). *Poverty: The Facts.* London, Child Poverty Action Group.
3 Rowntree, B. S. (1941). *Poverty and Progress.* London, Longmans, Green.
4 Townsend, P. (1979). *Poverty in the United Kingdom.* Harmondsworth, Penguin.
5 Council of Ministers, European Economic Community. (1981). *Final Report of the First Programme of Pilot Schemes and Studies to Combat Poverty.* Brussels, Commission of the European Communities.
6 Joseph, K. and Sumption, J. (1979). *Equality.* London, John Murray.
7 *Observer,* 14 May 1989: 15.
8 Church of England (1985). *Faith in the City.* London, Church House.
9 Townsend, P. (1979). 'Living with unemployment' in Walker, A. and Walker, C.

(eds) *The Growing Divide – A Social Audit 1979–1987*. London, Child Poverty Action Group.

10 Mack, J. and Lansley, S. (1985). *Poor Britain*. London, Allen & Unwin.

11 Mack, J. and Lansley, S. (1985). *ibid*.

12 Graham, H. (1984). *Women, Health and the Family*. Brighton, Wheatsheaf.

13 Piachaud, D. (1981). Children and Poverty, *Poverty Research Series*, no. 9, London, Child Poverty Action Group.

14 Bradshaw, J. and Morgan, J. (1987). *Budgeting on Benefit*. London, Family Policy Studies Centre.

15 Department of Health and Social Security, 1988 *Low Income Family Statistics, 1985*. London, HMSO.

16 House of Commons Social Service Committee (1990). *Income Support System and the Distribution of Income in 1987*. Study commissioned for the Institute for Fiscal Studies. London, HMSO.

17 Johnson, P. and Webb, S. (1989). *Counting People with Low Incomes: The Impact of Recent Changes*. London, Institute for Fiscal Studies.

18 Johnson, P. and Webb, S. (1990). *Poverty in Official Statistics: Two Reports*. London, Institute for Fiscal Studies.

19 Department of Social Security (1990). *Households Below Average Income Statistics*. London, Government Statistical Service.

20 Equal Opportunities Commission (1988). *Men and Women*. London, HMSO.

21 National Council for One-Parent Families (1988). *70th Annual Report*. London, National Council for One-Parent Families.

22 Millar, J. and Glendinning, C. (1989). *Women and Poverty*. Brighton, Wheatsheaf.

23 Pahl, J. (1980). 'Patterns of money management within marriage' *Journal of Social Policy*, vol. 9, 3: 313–35.

24 Quoted by Graham, H. (1984). op. cit.

25 Scott, H. (1984). 'Working your way up to the bottom', *The Feminisation of Poverty*. London, Pandora Press.

26 Lewis, J. and Piachaud, D. (1987). 'Women and poverty in the twentieth century', in Glendinning, C. and Millar, J. (eds) *Women and Poverty in Britain*. Brighton, Wheatsheaf.

27 Gordon, P. and Newnham, A. (1985). 'Passports to benefits?', *Racism in Social Security*. London, Child Poverty Action Group and the Runnymede Trust.

28 Becker, S. and MacPherson, S. (1988). op. cit.

29 Breadline Britain Survey (1984). See Mack, J. and Lansley, S. (1985). *Poor Britain*. London, Allen & Unwin.

30 Becker, S. (1988). 'Poverty awareness', in Becker, S. and MacPherson, S. *Public Issues, Private Pain*. London, Insight.

31 Taylor, D. (1987). 'Living with unemployment', in Walker, A. and Walker, C. (eds) *The Growing Divide – A Social Audit 1979–1987*. London, Child Poverty Action Group.

32 Department of Employment (1990). *Employment Gazette*, July 1990. London, HMSO.

33 Taylor, D. (1987). op. cit.

34 Department of Employment (1989). *Employment Gazette*, February 1989. London, HMSO.

35 Taylor, D. (1987). op. cit.

36 Department of Employment (1989). op. cit.

37 Glendinning, C. (1987). 'Impoverishing women', in Walker, A. and Walker, C. (eds) *The Growing Divide – A Social Audit 1979–1987*. London, Child Poverty Action Group.
38 Taylor, D. (1987). op. cit.
39 Cook, J. and Watt, S. (1987). 'Racism, women, and poverty', in Glendinning, C. and Millar, J. (eds) *Women and Poverty in Britain*. Brighton, Wheatsheaf.
40 Phizacklea, A. (1983). 'In the front line', in Phizacklea, A. (ed.) *One Way Ticket – Migration and Female Labour*. London, Routledge & Kegan Paul.
41 Berthoud, R. (1984). *The Reform of Supplementary Benefit*. London, Policy Studies Institute.
42 Oppenheim, C. (1990). *The Costs of a Child*. London, Child Poverty Action Group.
43 Walsh, A. and Lister, R. (1985). *Mothers' Life-Line: A Survey of How Women Use and Value Child Benefits*. London, Child Poverty Action Group.
44 Bidwell, S., Potter, T. and Rice, C. (1990). *The Growing Divide: Poverty, Health and Government Reform of the National Health Service*. Birmingham, West Midlands Low Pay Unit/West Midlands Health Service Monitoring Unit.
45 Winyard, S. and Pond, C. (1989). *Ten Years On: The Poor Decade*. London, Low Pay Unit.
46 Millar, J. and Glendinning, C. (1987). op. cit.
47 Brown, C. (1984). *Black and White Britain*. Third Policy Studies Institute Survey, London, PSI.
48 House of Commons *Hansard*, October 1988.
49 Quoted by Oppenheim, C. (1988). *Poverty: The Facts*. London, Child Poverty Action Group.
50 Smyth, M. and Robus, N. (1988). *The Financial Circumstances of Families with Disabled Children Living in Private Households*. OPCS Survey of Disability in Great Britain, Report No. 5. London, HMSO.
51 Martin, J. and White, A. (1988). *The Financial Circumstances of Disabled Adults Living in Private Households*. OPCS Survey of Disability in Great Britain, Report No. 2. London, HMSO.
52 Disability Alliance (1988). *Disability Rights Handbook*, 13th edition, April 1988–April 1989. Disability Alliance Education and Research Association.
53 Hill, J. (1988). *Changing Tax*. London, Child Poverty Action Group.

2 | POVERTY: THE HEALTH HAZARD

INTRODUCTION

Chapter 1 pointed to the scale of poverty and material deprivation in families with children in Britain. The fact that a growing number of families with children are forced to live in these circumstances means that those who are concerned with the welfare of families cannot afford to ignore the social and economic circumstances of their clients. The daily experience of 'doing without' not only brings material hardships but also the health costs of poverty. For health and welfare workers, the key question to be asked and answered is 'What are the links between poverty and health?'

The health costs of poverty have been documented in studies from as early as the 1830s and 1840s, when Chadwick carried out the first systematic investigation of the health effects of poverty.[1] This and other studies[2,3] have not only documented a clear association between poverty and health, they also point to clear health differences between social groups: between people of different social classes, between men and women, and between people of different ethnic groups. Whilst public-health measures and rises in living standards have done much to improve the health and life expectancy of the population, social inequalities in health persist. Moreover, these studies indicate that inequalities in health have not only persisted but have widened. The health status of poor social groups has failed to improve as fast as other groups.

Although studies have indicated a clear link between poverty and poor health, they have failed to address the nature of the link itself. Whilst the nature of the link between health and poverty is a crucial issue for field-workers, social research has been trying to address another (but related) question. It has been primarily concerned with the relationship between social position (social class, gender and 'race') and health. This focus on social position and health initially appears to be a major drawback. However, if we examine the data more closely, we can glean a lot of useful information about the health experiences of low-income groups. First, research on social position captures how inter-relating factors, such as income, housing and employment status affect health. For it is the whole complex of factors that make up people's lives that impact on their health. Second, social position is a good proxy measure for income and access to material resources. Focusing on working-class and Black people's experiences through social position provides a very approximate way of looking, at the macro level, how low income links with a cluster of disadvantages associated with poor health. An analysis of gender patterns extends our understanding by sharpening our appreciation of how paid and unpaid work patterns and conditions, not adequately reflected by social class, appear to be important. Furthermore, it reflects how complex these health patterns are. Poverty and low social position go hand in hand.

This chapter will examine the key question 'How does poverty affect health?' To attempt to answer this question the chapter will examine the following areas:

- *Patterns of health according to social position:* The chapter will use the wealth of data on social position and health to document how social class, gender, and 'race' are linked to both the income and income support patterns we observed in chapter 1 and the health status of poor families.
- *The relationship between income and health:* Examining how income can help us to understand what it is about social position that shapes people's health status. Here the chapter will focus on how income determines access to key health resources, and offer some tentative reasons why social class inequalities have widened, contrary to popular expectations.
- *The processes by which poverty affects health:* Here the chapter will draw together the information we have on poverty and health into a framework which helps us to understand how poverty shapes health in complex ways. The framework emphasizes three inter-linking processes: physiological, psychological, and behavioural.[4]

This information helps us to question many current beliefs about the causes of ill health among low-income groups. It illustrates that the health of poor families is not within their personal control and is the outcome of low income and poor access to health resources.

PATTERNS OF HEALTH BY SOCIAL POSITION

People vary in health as they vary in every other aspect of their lives. When we examine the area of inequalities in health we are generally focusing not on health differences that are the outcome of natural genetic variation or personality, but health differences that are shaped by social and economic factors. The concept of health inequalities carries with it the idea that health differences due to social and economic disadvantage are unjust. At a meeting on social justice, the World Health Organization (1984)[5] stated that in health terms: 'everyone should have the same opportunity to attain the highest level of health and, more pragmatically, none should be unduly disadvantaged.'

Indicators of health and illness tell us clearly that some groups are disadvantaged, with some groups experiencing far worse health than others. Measuring this difference in health experience is almost as problematical as measuring poverty. It involves measures of health status and measures of inequality. In trying to measure the first of these concepts, health, there has been a trend away from medical models of health that equate health with the absence of disease, towards broader models that encompass physical, psychological and social well-being:

The World Health Organization (1978) defines health as 'a state of complete physical, psychological, and social well-being and not merely the absence of disease and infirmity'.[6]

The Royal College of General Practitioners (1972) defines health as 'a satisfactory adjustment of the individual to the environment'.[7]

It has been difficult to develop indicators of health that reflect this new thinking. Concepts such as 'well-being' and 'adjustment to the environment' are very difficult to measure in a meaningful statistical way. The most reliable measures of health are, in fact, measures of ill health that stem from a medical model. Whilst most fieldworkers are happier with a broader, social model of health, mortality (death) rates and morbidity (illness) rates remain the most used, surrogate indicators of health for practical reasons. The Office of Populations Census and Surveys (OPCS) has provided statistical information on mortality and aspects of morbidity for years. Reflecting the shift from a medical (health and the absence of disease) approach to health to a more social model, there has been a proliferation of new measures and surveys that aim to assess the more subjective elements of physical, psychological and social health. Important examples are the *Health and Lifestyles Survey*,[8] the *General Health Questionnaire*[9] and the *Nottingham Health Profile*.[10] Although intended to complement rather than replace the traditional indicators that provide hard data, many of these new tools appear promising as alternative measures of health status. They will become more useful as comparisons over time become available, and they begin to provide information on a range of health factors that have not been available before. From necessity this chapter will rely on OPCS data predominantly, complementing these data with data from the newer types of studies where appropriate.

New measures of health and illness suggest that health is related to a host of social factors, including education, occupation, income, housing tenure and conditions, car ownership and environmental conditions. A person's relationship to these social factors appears to be strongly related to his/her social class, gender and 'race'. Differences in health experience and life expectancy between people of different social classes, between people of different ethnic groups, and between men and women are the most distinctive form of health inequalities in Britain today. The next three sub-sections will discuss each of these forms of health inequality in turn.

SOCIAL CLASS AND HEALTH

Social class is the most widely used indicator of the social and economic circumstances of individuals. It is used to distinguish groups who are thought to share a common way of life and a common level of resources. Social class is a central concept in the study of health inequalities as it is used to show how social and economic circumstances are related to the health experiences, and expectations, of individuals. Although a number of factors, such as income, type of housing and education play a part in determining a person's social class, occupation has generally been thought to be the best indicator of socio-economic status. Occupation does not simply indicate type of work but also implies working conditions, level of pay, access to fringe benefits and, therefore, access to other resources. Thus it can be said to also be related to income, housing status and education. The most common social classification used in British surveys is based on the Registrar-General's classification of occupations (see table 2.1).

When people are allocated to a social class, their gender and position in the household determine where they are placed. In most health studies, while men's social class is directly related to their occupation, women's and children's social class is indirectly ascribed:

☐ Men are allocated a social class according to their own occupation.

☐ Married women are ascribed the social class of their husband.

☐ Children in two-parent families are ascribed the social class of their father.

☐ Single women living alone, or with their children, are allocated a social class according to their own occupation.

While the Registrar-General's social-class classification based on occupation is thought to give a general guide to social position, it is probably a less accurate measure than it was. Increasing home ownership, second incomes, single parenthood, and unemployment cut across the traditional

TABLE 2.1   Registrar-General's classification of social class

Social class		Examples of occupations
I	Professional	Lawyer, doctor,
II	Intermediate	Teacher, nurse, manager
III(NM)	Skilled non-manual	Typist, shop assistant
III(M)	Skilled manual	Miner, cook, electrician
IV	Semi-skilled manual	Farm worker, packer
V	Unskilled manual	Cleaner, labourer

relationship between a man's occupation and his family resources.[11] There is some concern that traditional measures based on occupation do not accurately reflect the social status and experiences of all groups:

 Some groups are poorly described by measures of social class based on occupations, for example, those who have never had a job, those who do not have a job now and married women who are classified according to their husband's social class.

 The Registrar-General's classification is based on a hierarchy that reflects the traditional status of male occupations. It does not always accurately reflect the status or experiences associated with women's occupations.

 It ascribes to all members of the same family the same social class. Thus it fails to recognize that some members of a family may experience poorer social and economic circumstances than others.

Social-class measures do not reflect that social class experiences are different for Black people and white people, just as they are for men and women.

Despite the limitations of social-class classifications based on measures of occupation, the Registrar-General's classification is used extensively. It has provided data on social class and mortality since 1921 and reveals a vast amount about how dimensions of social class relate to health. As the evidence on health inequalities is extensive, the next section will attempt only to highlight some of the key areas and general trends in health inequalities.

At almost every age, people in the poorer social classes (social classes IV and V), have higher rates of illness and death than people in wealthier social classes (social classes I and II). This pattern of inequalities is most marked in the first year of life and least marked in adolescence and early adulthood.

Statistics on death in the first year of life are thought to be one of the most sensitive indicators of the health of the population. Perinatal mortality rates (all stillbirths and deaths occurring in the first week of life) and postneonatal mortality rates (deaths occurring between twenty-eight days and one year) are the most commonly used statistics. Because perinatal mortality rates are now low overall, there is a concern as to whether they can be used reliably as a health measure. None the less, despite this note of caution, they do point to divergent patterns between social classes. This mortality gap between social classes has remained fairly constant since the early 1970s and persists even when factors which increase the risk of perinatal mortality, such as maternal age and family size, are controlled for. The mortality gap between classes is even greater in the postneonatal period than the perinatal period but, like the perinatal mortality rate, there has been very little change in the size of the gap since the mid-1970s.

 In 1986, babies born to social class IV and V families were 148 per cent more likely to die in the perinatal period than babies born to social class I and II families.[12]

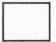 In 1986, babies born to parents in social classes IV and V had a 178-per-cent greater chance of dying in the postneonatal period than babies of social class I and II parents.[13]

Low birth weight is also clearly associated with social class. It is thought to be associated with parental poverty and a poor material environment, rather than the quality of medical care. Although poverty and the poorer material environment of working-class babies contribute to the increased incidence of premature death in the perinatal period, it is not clear as yet, exactly how big their contribution is.

Two-thirds of all low-birth-weight babies are born to working-class mothers.[14]

For children aged 1–15 years deaths also vary clearly by social class, though less widely than in the postneonatal period. For individual causes of death, class differences in mortality rates appear to be steepest for accidents and infections, and lowest or absent for deaths from childhood cancer.[15] It is thought that social-class gradients in childhood mortality are steepest where environmental factors play a part. These steep class gradients are thought to reflect working-class children's experience of poverty and conditions such as poor housing and lack of safe play areas.[16] The childhood death rate from accidents, the largest single cause of death in childhood, is a clear example of how living in a poor physical environment, without the resources to make it safe, has serious consequences for the health of children. Chapter 4 illustrates how poverty and poor housing conditions go hand in hand, and how together they impact on the lives of parents and children.

 The mortality rate for all causes of death tells us that children aged 1–15, from social classes IV and V, are twice as likely to die as their counterparts from social classes I and II.[17]

Although mortality rates are thought to be the most accurate, surrogate measure of health status, it is also important to quantify the amount of illness that children suffer. Comparing morbidity (illness) between different social groups is more problematic than comparing mortality. Most morbidity statistics are based on reported or identified ill health and are gathered in studies that record self-reporting (or, in the case of a child, parental reporting of symptoms), or medical consultation/hospital admission rates. These types of data depend, first, on an individual's interpreting his/her symptoms as illness and reporting them; second, the doctor or researcher's recording these symptoms as ill health; and, third, in the case of consultation/admission rates, the person's seeking medical help. Yet research has shown that self-reporting of illness and help-seeking behaviour are related to perceptions about the meaning of illness, knowledge about the symptoms and ability or desire to seek help. These aspects of health behaviour have been shown to be influenced by social disadvantage, poverty, low educational attainment and wider cultural factors. It appears that studies that rely solely on self-reporting of illness or use of services are likely to underestimate morbidity in manual social classes.

Despite the fact that morbidity data are difficult to interpret clearly, they do generally confirm the same picture as the mortality statistics. Social-class differences in health do exist, with children from manual social classes generally experiencing more illness than children from social classes I and II:

 Large-scale longitudinal studies show that children from manual classes suffer more respiratory infections and diseases, ear infections, and squints, and are likely to be of shorter stature than their counterparts in non-manual classes.[18,19]

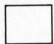 Children from manual social classes are also more likely to have less healthy teeth. In 1983, children from manual social classes had twice as many decayed teeth as their counterparts.[20]

The health of adults as well as children is linked to their social position. *Whilst class inequalities in health are narrower in adulthood than childhood, the statistics tell us that death rates are far higher for poorer classes than richer classes:*

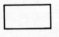 For the years 1979–83, the mortality rate was twice as high for adults in social class V as for adults in social class I.[21]

 In 1981, if manual workers had had the same death rates as non-manual workers in the age range 17–74 years, there would have been 42,000 fewer deaths during that year.[22]

Almost all major killer diseases affect manual classes more than non-manual classes. This suggests that wider socio-economic factors are operating consistently in a way that increases mortality rates among those in social classes IV and V. Those who wish to examine mortality rates by specific causes of death will find analyses by Marmot and McDowall (1986)[23] or Townsend *et al.* (1987)[24] useful. What is striking is that the diseases that were once thought of as 'diseases of affluence', such as coronary heart disease and cancer, are now more accurately described as diseases of social and economic disadvantage and poverty.

Not only are adults in manual classes more likely to die from major diseases, they also suffer more ill health. Blaxter (1987) argues that morbidity rates and indicators of general health status are becoming more important indicators of health inequality now that people are living longer but suffering more chronic and degenerative diseases.[25]

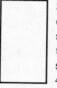 Surveys indicate that inequalities in health experience between classes still exist: the gradient is steepest for limiting longstanding illness, with unskilled manual classes reporting rates that are double those of professional classes, less steep for longstanding illness and only evident for acute illness reporting at age 45 and over.[26,27]

The *Health and Lifestyles Survey* indicates that, if income, rather than social class, is used as the variable, the differences in health experiences become clearer still. Those with lower incomes report higher rates of symptoms and are far more likely to assess their own health as poor, compared to those on higher incomes.[28]

People from poorer social classes use health services more frequently than richer social classes, but not as much as would be expected from their higher levels of illness. The pattern of general-practitioner consultation rates and use of preventative services do not follow the same social-class-related patterns as death and illness rates.

'RACE', ETHNICITY AND HEALTH

A further important and inter-linking dimension of social position is 'race' and ethnicity. It has been shown that focusing on people's ethnic status, particularly the experience of racism, provides a very illuminating way of looking at the distribution of social disadvantage and poor health between social groups. In chapter 1 it became evident that ethnic status shapes a person's access to material and social resources. The data indicate that minority ethnic groups, particularly Black groups, have poorer access to health resources including income, employment, good housing and living conditions, transport and education than other groups. A growing body of research evidence clearly indicates that individual and institutional racial discrimination results in minority ethnic groups receiving a small and unjust share of material resources.[29] People from minority ethnic groups, particularly Black people, are more likely to be unemployed, or be in low-paid jobs, live in poor housing and live in areas that lack adequate social and educational resources than white people. Black people share the disadvantages of white working-class people and more.

The evidence suggests that racial differences in health clearly reflect differences in social environments between Black and minority ethnic and white groups. However, some people still tend to blame health differences between majority and minority ethnic groups on genetic differences or cultural differences or deficits. The evidence suggests that racial groups are genetically similar in their susceptibility to disease, with the exception of a few specific diseases (for example, sickle cell anaemia and thalassaemia). The lifestyles and health choices of Black and minority ethnic groups are sometimes viewed as unhealthy, backward, bizarre and inferior to those of white groups. For example, the vegetarian diet of Asian families is frequently seen as the root of health problems such as rickets and heart disease, although there is little concrete evidence that these diseases can be explained in this way.

Measuring racial inequalities in health, like the measurement of social-class inequalities, is fraught with problems. Overall, the problems inherent in 'race' and health data tend to underestimate the extent of inequalities and fail adequately to describe the types of health problems and experiences of Black and minority ethnic groups:

 Ethnicity is often inferred from information about people's country of birth. As a result we know little about the health status and experiences of Black and minority ethnic groups born in Britain who now constitute a growing proportion (40 per cent)[30] of the minority ethnic community.

Some research studies are based on interviewer-ascribed ethnic origin. This is likely to introduce biases into studies.

Research studies have tended to concentrate on diseases and health problems that interest doctors, such as schizophrenia and rickets, rather than on the everyday health problems experienced by Black and minority ethnic groups themselves.

Measures do not reflect that racial inequalities are the outcome of social class position and gender as well as 'race'.

The main differences between different ethnic groups appear to be related to differences in access to material resources. Beginning with the early years of life, OPCS data on outcomes of pregnancy by mother's country of birth allow us to look at the effect of ethnicity on perinatal and infant mortality, and birth weight:

 Mortality rates are consistently higher and have reduced less quickly for babies of mothers born in the New Commonwealth and Pakistan than for mothers born in the UK.[31]

FIGURE 2.1 Standardized mortality rates (ages 20–49) by sex and country of birth compared to UK-born adults, 1979–83

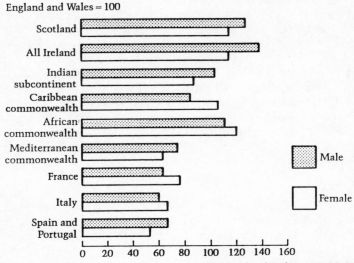

Source: OPCS (1990). Mortality among Immigrants in England and Wales, 1979-83, Balarajan, R. and Bulusu, L. in Britten, M. (ed.) (1990). *Mortality and Geography*. Series DS 9. London, HMSO.

Studies of local populations have tried to unravel the cause of these disparities around childbirth. Low birth weight and congenital malformations are the most important causes of perinatal mortality. Although perinatal mortality rates are sometimes thought to reflect the quality of maternity care available to mothers, low birth weight is more closely associated with poverty and material deprivation. Studies of pregnancy outcomes in mothers born outside England and Wales have not assessed the influence of material deprivation and poverty on perinatal mortality rates. It is likely that these rates can partly be attributed to the social and economic conditions of minority ethnic groups.

The first comprehensive study of the mortality rates of adults born abroad was carried out as late as the early 1980s by Marmot *et al.* (1984).[32] This and more recent research show a mixed picture, with mortality rates differing between people born in England and Wales and people born abroad, and between different ethnic groups for different diseases. Figure 2.1 shows how mortality rates differ by country of birth for those born outside England and Wales, compared to those adults born inside England and Wales.

Mortality rates differ for specific diseases according to country of birth. For example, while the death rate from coronary heart disease is highest for those born in the Indian subcontinent, death rates from hypertension and strokes are higher for people born in Afro-Caribbean countries. Deaths from cancer are low in those from African countries and the Indian subcontinent.[33] Tuberculosis, diabetes and liver cancer cause higher death rates in adults born in the Indian subcontinent and Afro-Caribbean countries, while the same group has lower death rates from obstructive lung diseases than people born in England and Wales.[34]

Statistical data on the mental health of Britain's minority ethnic and Black population are just as patchy as data on physical health and subject to many of the same problems. Studies indicate that Black people born outside the UK are more likely to be admitted to psychiatric hospitals,[35] be diagnosed as suffering from a psychotic illness[36] and receive physical treatments[37] (such as major tranquillizers and electroconvulsive therapy) than UK-born adults. Patterns of mental health among Britain's Black and white population will be discussed in chapter 5.

GENDER AND HEALTH

So far we have discussed the effect of social class and ethnic status on health without referring to the fact that mortality and morbidity patterns may be different for men and women. Although social class has an important influence on health, gender also exerts an influence on the duration and quality of life that is independent of social class. For Black women, the experience of racism exerts an influence on their health that is over and above the experiences of white women. It is to these important aspects of health inequality that this chapter now turns.

When we examine gender inequalities in health, we are generally looking at the effect that men's and women's different working and living conditions exert on health. In chapter 1 we saw how the social position of women determines their access to income and income support. Woman's reduced access to the labour market, her family structure and her role as primary carer in the family are crucial factors. Moreover, for women, their access to material resources may be further restricted by their ethnic group. The data in chapter 1 suggest that Black women and their children suffer the worst social and economic disadvantage. Before going on to examine gender specific patterns of health, it should be noted that some of the gender differences reflect biological differences and not social differences. Cancers and disorders of the male and female reproductive organs, such as cancer of the breast, ovary and testicle, fall into this category. Women's capacity to conceive and give birth to children appears to be related to specific health problems and illnesses.

The relationship between gender and health is more complex than that of social class and health. Gender does not operate in the same unidimensional way. Instead, cross-cutting forces appear to be in operation, protecting and undermining the health of men and women in different ways.[38]

Measuring gender differences, like 'race' and social class differences, is not free from difficulties. It is useful to note some of the common concerns:

Women's social inequalities in health have not been mapped as extensively as those of men.

 Women's social and economic environment is not adequately reflected by social class.

 Measures of gender differences in health often fail to reflect that Black and white women have different social and economic experiences.

Mortality and morbidity rates for women generally follow similar class gradients to those of men when women are classified according to the social class of the male head of household. Although studies which have examined social-class inequalities in health in relation to women's own jobs have found striking inequalities under certain conditions, the picture is confusing. For example, cancers of the ovary and breast are more common among women from richer social classes than poorer classes.[39] However, this may be a reflection of differences in childbearing patterns. Any analysis of women's health patterns by their own occupation only highlights the need for more research, and the need to develop a social-class measure that reflects the nature of their own unpaid and paid employment.

The general pattern of health which characterizes the difference between the sexes is that 'men die and women are sick'. Men have higher death rates than women at every age, in a ratio of 2:1.[40] Some researchers have suggested that differences in mortality rates between the sexes can be explained in terms of differences in behaviour;[41] but a more favoured explanation is that they reflect differences in social and economic conditions for men and women.[42] It is evident that differences in mortality rates between men and women are narrowing for some causes of death. However, some of this narrowing is due to rising death rates from certain diseases, such as lung cancer, among women.

The causes of death, as well as rates of death, vary between men and women:

 Deaths from accidents and violence are more common among males in childhood and early adulthood.[43]

 In middle age, circulatory diseases are the commonest cause of death for men, while women are more likely to die from cancer, particularly of the breast or lung.[44]

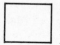 Men are more prone than women to die or be seriously injured at work. But women's occupations have their own patterns of hazards, for instance back injuries are common among nurses.[45]

Deaths from suicide are higher among men, particularly among men of social class V. More than half of these deaths are thought to be related to unemployment rather than psychiatric illness.[46]

If we consider morbidity differences between the sexes, the pattern is reversed. *Although women live longer than men, they suffer more chronic and acute illnesses.*

 Studies of mental illness indicate that women consistently suffer higher rates of neurotic and depressive illnesses than men.[47]

 Women are more likely than men to assess their own health as poor or very poor.[48]

There is some debate about the meaning of these sex differences in the rates of mental illness. Chapter 5 will discuss possible explanations for these differences.

THE RELATIONSHIP BETWEEN HEALTH AND POVERTY

An examination of health differences according to social position has reminded us that social inequalities in health still persist. People from manual social classes, women and Black and minority ethnic groups have the highest death and illness rates. There have been many attempts to explain the existence of health inequalities. Genetic theories fail to provide an adequate explanation for those differences, although genetic factors clearly explain some individual differences within groups. It has also been suggested that social-class differences are the outcome of natural and social selection: the process whereby those with the poorest health move down the social scale, whilst those with good health move up the social scale. Although there is some evidence that this process exists at younger ages, it cannot explain the overall differences in health that exist between social groups. The data on social position and health suggest that a whole complex of inter-related social and economic factors impact on people's health. In the last decade several researchers have been trying to discover what it is about social position that influences patterns of health by concentrating on the role that income plays in health.

As we saw earlier, the three elements of social position – class, 'race' and gender – interlink to determine an individual's and a family's degree of access to income and, therefore, access to the material resources that are important for health. To examine the relationship between health and income, it is useful to begin by looking at this relationship from the macro level, and then to move on in the next section to examine, at the micro level, the processes by which low income is likely to shape family health.

INCOME AS A HEALTH RESOURCE

Household income is the greatest determinant of living standards. It touches every part of family life. It influences where a family lives (and hence the family's degree of exposure to environmental hazards), access to space, leisure, work, educational facilities and health-care resources. Income influences the quality of housing and hence the family's degree of exposure to the diseases associated with damp and cold. It influences how much money is available for food, fuel and clothing and thus the body's capacity to regenerate and resist infection. The total of these determine a family's degree of domestic comfort and contributes to their sense of physical, social and emotional well-being. In this way, a focus on income shows us how the exposure to one health hazard, low income, increases the chance of exposure to other health hazards such as inadequate diet, poor housing and lack of social and recreational facilities.

Blaxter (1990), [49] analysing data from the *Health and Lifestyles Survey*, has attempted to ascertain to what extent social-class health differences reflect differences in income. She found that the apparent strong association between social class and health was primarily one of income and health. Wilkinson's research (1986)[50] has also highlighted the important influence of income on health. Moreover, this study of the relationship between income and mortality has begun to shed some light on why social inequalities in health persist and have widened. By focusing on income, rather than social position, he has shown that changes in income levels correlate with changes in health. The box that follows describes Wilkinson's main findings:

An analysis of occupational incomes has shown that those occupations that enjoyed the fastest rises in income also experienced the fastest fall in death rates, while those that had the slowest rise in income had the slowest fall in death rates.[51]

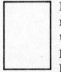

National evidence on the effect of the changing value of state retirement pensions on death rates illustrates a correlation between death rates of older adults and the real value of state pensions. As the real value of retirement pensions has declined, pensioners' death rates have risen.[52]

This evidence helps to explain the controversial health statistics that show a widening of social-class differences in health, despite rises in absolute income and living standards. Wilkinson suggests that the post-war widening of mortality rates between social classes is related to the trend in relative poverty.[53] Since as early as 1921, the trend in social-class mortality differences has matched the pattern of the trend in relative poverty. A decline in the number of people suffering the worst poverty in the period 1921–50 was accompanied by a narrowing of social-class differences in death rates. Around the year 1950, the proportion of the population living in relative poverty was at its lowest level since 1921, with only 8 per cent of the population in poverty. By 1987, the number of people living in poverty had risen to 28 per cent of the population (see chapter 1). This rise in the level of relative poverty was accompanied by a corresponding widening of death

FIGURE 2.2   Example of curvilinear relationship between poverty and health

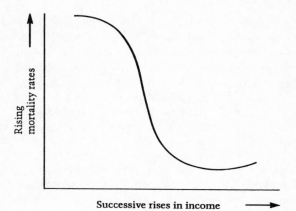

rates by social class. Over this period the death rates for social classes I and II reduced faster than those for social classes IV and V. The atypical narrowing of death rates for young women since 1975 may well be related to the increase in women's economic activity, and the relative improvement in women's pay after the Equal Pay Act.

This evidence reinforces the view that we need to work with a relative view of poverty. With overall rises in living standards over the century, death rates for the poor have not fallen as fast as death rates for the rich. Being healthy appears to require more than an absolute level of income to stay alive. It requires a level of income which allows families to enjoy similar living standards and participate in a similar way as families with higher incomes.

Both Blaxter's and Wilkinson's data suggest that the relationship between income and health is unlikely to be one that runs in a straight line: where increases in income bring successive health gains. The relationship is more likely to be a curvilinear line, where successive rises in income bring health gains only to a certain point, after which there may be no further gains, or even losses. Thus those groups with very high incomes may have poorer health than those with incomes that are moderately high. Figure 2.2 illustrates the probable shape of the relationship between poverty and health.

Further research is needed to establish the exact shape of the curve. It is particularly important to find out at what point, if at all, successive gains in income are no longer associated with positive gains in health. Moreover, if the shape of the curve is curvilinear, increases in income among those on the lowest incomes would be expected to have a dramatic effect on mortality rates.

PROCESSES BY WHICH POVERTY AFFECTS HEALTH

To develop an insight into the relationship between health and poverty, we need to look beyond national mortality and morbidity data to the micro level: to the level of the individual, and the processes by which poverty may influence a person's susceptibility to a disease or condition. Although we have only limited knowledge of how the various processes operate, it is possible to examine the general nature of these processes by separating them. Whilst separating out these processes is creating artificial distinctions between processes which are, in reality, intertwined, the exercise is useful for two main reasons. First, it enables us to see that more than one process is at work. The evidence suggests that at least three main processes need to be examined if we are to understand the way in which poverty shapes family health and family health care:[54] physiological, psychological, and behavioural processes. Second, it reminds us that poverty affects every aspect of health, from physical, mental and social health through to health behaviour. These three main processes will be discussed in turn in the next three sub-sections.

PHYSIOLOGICAL PROCESSES

The most well-researched and understood way in which poverty affects health can be described as a physiological process. Poor access to material resources for health and greater exposure to health hazards that result from poverty directly harm the body, depriving it of basic necessities for life and reducing its ability to cope with stresses and infections. This is probably the process that is easiest to understand, as it fits in well with our understanding of a medical model of disease causation. This process is exemplified in studies that have sought to show the direct relationship between poor diet and ill health, and poor housing conditions and ill health.

An inadequate diet directly affects children's growth and development, the health of pregnant women and is related to diseases such as coronary heart disease. Research indicates that low income restricts food choices and limits the quality of food consumed.[55] Low-income families are more likely to live in damp and cold housing conditions. Platt et al.'s[56] research has indicated that exposure to damp and mouldy living conditions has a direct effect on health. Allergic reactions to mould growth are likely to explain the higher levels of respiratory infections, tiredness and fevers found among people, particularly children, living in these conditions. This study also highlights how physical symptoms of illness link to emotional behaviours. Physical symptoms triggered off by the mould appear to cause increased irritability and unhappiness in children, and 'bad nerves' in parents. These psychological processes, in turn, shape behaviour: temper outbursts in children or smoking habits among parents.

From this we can see that the physical effects of poverty are also an indirect cause and consequence of psychological stress associated with the daily experience of breadline living. Stress is associated with a number of physical-illness symptoms – tiredness, muscle pains, and palpitations – as well as actual ill health, for example, gastro-intestinal disorders.

An understanding of how poverty affects health physically is important. However, on its own, it fails to illustrate how the health effects of poverty are not the consequences simply of choices about behaviour and lifestyle, but the outcome of factors that shape behaviour indirectly. To appreciate fully the complexity of the relationship it is necessary to examine how poverty affects health through psychological and behavioural processes.

PSYCHOLOGICAL PROCESSES

Poverty takes its toll on mental well-being. Money and high social status buy choice and influence to solve problems. Poverty, on the other hand, allows little scope to cope with either the day-in, day-out stress of limited access to material resources, or with stressful life-events such as bereavement, loss of employment or marriage breakdown. Not only does poverty appear to increase the number of stressful life-events for families, it also appears to militate against the successful resolution of that stress. Parenting on low income appears to be associated with high levels of stress and depression. The social position of low-income families means that parents are less likely to have the physical resources, the emotional support from confiding relationships or a level of social support that helps them to cope with the additional pressures that parenting in poverty brings.

Poverty brings with it relative powerlessness and lack of control over events. Fisher's theory of 'locus of control' suggests that those people who believe that they have some control over the source of stress may be less at risk of developing a sense of helplessness and depressive illnesses than those who feel they have no control.[57] Beliefs about whether events are within one's personal control depend on previous experiences. The daily experience of poverty does little to foster a sense of 'being in control'. Moreover, studies of the experiences of poverty, some of which will be described in future chapters, have documented how the very nature of being dependent on social-security benefits prevents individuals exercising control. For example, the timing and arrival of social-security payments are often out of the control of individuals and dependent on the efficiency of social security staff and the postal system. Lack of opportunity to exercise control over one's life and dependence on others for high levels of financial and material support also work against feelings of positive self-esteem. Those who lack the personal or social resources to deal with stress and conflict may develop methods of coping, such as drugs abuse, heavy drinking or smoking, that are less satisfactory and likely to be damaging to physical health. Here we can begin to see how psychological processes not only interact with physiological processes, but also behavioural processes.

BEHAVIOURAL PROCESSES

Our health is affected by our behaviour. Behaviours – such as eating, smoking, drinking – and leisure habits, use of health services and social relationships with others affect our physical and mental health. Different behaviour patterns account for some of the differences in health experiences between social groups. The idea that behaviour is within the control of the individual underlies much health and welfare work and many of the government's health promotion programmes. The poor health of many low-income groups is frequently explained in terms of their unhealthy patterns of behaviour. As a consequence, the poor are chastised and urged to act more responsibly by choosing healthier lifestyles and behaviours. Research and theory from the social sciences have sought to draw attention to the limitations of this model. This research has highlighted that behaviour does not occur in a social vacuum. It is shaped by social and economic circumstances. Researchers who have looked at the experiences of families in poverty have illustrated how low income constrains behaviour. For example, low income confines the type of food that low-income families can purchase and therefore the amount of nutrients individuals can eat.[58] Studies of the attitudes of low-income families to food indicate that they are knowledgeable about food and would prefer to eat a healthy diet.[59] Studies of the cost of a healthy diet show that whilst low-income families would prefer a healthier diet, their food choices, particularly the choices of those dependent on social-security benefits, are severely limited by their incomes.[60] They are unable to buy the foods recommended by healthy-eating programmes. In this way, income clearly shapes behaviour (see chapter 3).

In the area of food choices and other areas of behaviour, poverty also affects health by not only reducing a family's access to health resources, but by placing them in a situation where they have to make health choices that serve to protect one aspect of health, or the health of another family member, whilst undermining another aspect of health or the health of another person. These health choices are often classed as reckless or irresponsible behaviour but appear to act as a mechanism for coping with some of the stress and hardships of poverty. For example, women in low-income families appear to continue to smoke as a way of coping with the tensions of bringing up children in poverty, even though they can least afford to smoke and know the personal health costs. Bottle feeding and the early introduction of solids are other examples of behaviours that serve to protect the health of some family members, in this case the mental health of mothers, whilst appearing to be irrational decisions to other people. In this sense, behaviour often determines the nature of the physiological and psychological processes that affect health in poverty.

Physiological, psychological and behavioural processes appear to interact in a complex way to determine the health status of families. For families in poverty, income, the key resource for health, appears to be the major factor that determines to which health hazards families are exposed.

CONCLUSION AND IMPLICATIONS FOR PRACTICE

This chapter has documented the poor health of groups living in adverse social and economic circumstances. The arguments in favour of improving the health experience and life expectancy of families in poverty have been well voiced, with a consensus that acknowledges the benefits both for the individual and society as a whole. Yet paradoxically the outcome of many health-promotion programmes has been an improvement in the health of the rich, therefore achieving results in inverse proportion to the distribution of ill health in the population. The fact that health promotion programmes have frequently failed to improve the health of the poor and have had the effect of widening inequalities in health is the consequence of preventive health and social-welfare programmes that fail to take into account the nature of the relationship between poverty and ill health. To adopt an approach, at fieldwork level up to policy-making level, that ignores the relationship between health, income and social position is 'as unscientific as to ignore the evidence of the relationship between nutritional factors and disease'.[61]

This chapter has adopted an approach that focuses on health and poverty by focusing on the role of income in health. This is an important but under-developed area of research. By using the research evidence on the link between social position and health, we have been able to document the relationship between social class, 'race', gender and health. Focusing on income has helped us to begin to discover what it is about social position that determines health. Income is a key resource that determines access to many other important health resources. Social position and income are closely related. People in low social classes, women and minority ethnic groups are likely to have the lowest incomes and the poorest health.

To understand the nature of the relationship between health and poverty it is useful to draw on the framework that shows which causative processes come into play. A framework that illustrates how physiological, psycho-logical and behavioural processes come into play explains the effect of phenomena other than poverty. It is a particularly useful framework to use in any attempt to explain the links between poverty and health as it avoids simplistic explanations that fail to take into account the relationship between the material and social conditions of people's lives and health behaviour. Moreover, it places the health and poverty debate firmly in the arena of social policy, rather than leaving it solely in the arena of health education. The reduction of inequalities in health will be achieved by a fundamental redistribution in wealth and significant rises in income and access to other material resources, such as good housing for low-income groups rather than better health-education programmes that focus on individual behaviour.

The following chapters will examine some specific dimensions of poverty – food poverty, poor housing and the stress of breadline living – to illustrate how poverty affects the health of those who experience it.

REFERENCES

1 Chadwick, E. (1842). *Report on the Sanitary Conditions of the Labouring Population of Great Britain*. Reprinted by Edinburgh University Press (1965).
2 Townsend, P. and Davidson, N. (eds) (1982). *Inequalities in Health*. Harmondsworth, Penguin.
3 Whitehead, M. (1987). *The Health Divide*. London, Health Education Council.
4 British Medical Association (1987). *Deprivation and Ill-Health*. London, British Medical Association.
5 World Health Organization (1984). *Report of the Working Group on Concepts and Principles in Health Promotion*. Copenhagen.
6 World Health Organization (1978). *Primary Health Care: Report of the International Conference of Primary Health Care*. Alma-Ata, 1978. Geneva, WHO.
7 Royal College of General Practitioners (1972). *The Future General Practitioner*. London, Royal College of General Practitioners.
8 Cox, B. D., *et al.* (1987). *The Health and Lifestyles Survey*. Cambridge, Health Promotion Research Trust.
9 Goldberg, D. P. (1972). *The Detection of Psychiatric Illness by Questionnaire*. Oxford, Oxford University Press.
10 Hunt, S. and McEwen, J. (1986). 'The development of a subjective health indicator' *Sociology of Health and Illness*, 2: 231–46.
11 Townsend, P., Phillimore, P. and Beattie, A. (1987). *Health and Deprivation, Inequality and the North*. London, Routledge.
12 Whitehead, M. (1987). op. cit.
13 Whitehead, M. (1987). op. cit.
14 Smith, A. and Jacobson, B. (1988). *The Nation's Health, A Strategy for the 1990s*. London, King's Fund.
15 Office of Populations, Censuses and Surveys (1988). *Occupational Mortality: Childhood Supplement 1979–80, 1982–83*. London, HMSO.
16 Blaxter, M. (1982). *The Health of Children*. London, Heinemann Educational Books.
17 Office of Populations, Censuses and Surveys (1988). op. cit.
18 Davie, R., Butler, N. and Goldstein, H. (1972). *From Birth to Seven*. London, Longman.
19 Tanner, J. M. (1986). 'Physical development' *British Medical Bulletin*, vol. 42, 2: 131–8.
20 Todd, J. E. and Todd, D. (1985). *Children's Dental Health in the UK, 1983*. London, HMSO.

21 Office of Populations, Censuses and Surveys (1986). *Occupational Mortality: Decennial Supplement 1979–80, 1982–83*. London, HMSO.
22 Smith, A. and Jacobson, B. (1988). op. cit.
23 Marmot, M. G. and McDowall, M. E. (1986). 'Mortality decline and widening social inequalities' *Lancet*, ii: 274–6.
24 Townsend, P. *et al.* (1987). op. cit.
25 Blaxter, M. (1987). 'A comparison of measures of inequality in morbidity' in Fox, A. (ed) *Inequalities in Health in Europe*. Aldershot, Gower.
26 Office of Populations, Censuses and Surveys (1989). *General Household Survey, 1987*. London, HMSO.
27 Cox, B. D., *et al.* (1987). op. cit.
28 Blaxter, M. (1990). op. cit.
29 Grimsley, M. and Bhat, A. (1988). 'Health', in Bhat, A. *et al.* (eds), *Britain's Black Population*. 2nd edition, Aldershot, Gower.
30 Office of Populations, Censuses and Surveys (1989). *Labour Force Survey, 1987*. London, HMSO.
31 Britton, M. (1989). 'Mortality and geography', OPCS, *Population Trends*, no. 56: 16–23.
32 Marmot, M., Adelstein, A. and Bulusu, L. (1983). 'Immigrant mortality in England and Wales' *Population Trends*, 33: 13–17.
33 Balarajah, R. and Bulusu, L. (1990). 'Mortality among immigrants in England and Wales', Britten, M. (ed.) *Mortality and Geography*, Series DS no. 9. London, HMSO.
34 Marmot, M. G. *et al.* (1983). op. cit.
35 Dean, G., Walsh, D., Downing, H. *et al.* (1981). 'First admissions of native-born and immigrants to psychiatric hospitals in South-East England, 1976' *British Journal of Psychiatry*, vol. 139: 506–12.
36 Cochrane, R. (1977). Cited in Grimsley, M. and Bhat, A. (1988). op. cit.
37 Donovan, J. (1984). 'Ethnicity and health: a research review' *Social Science and Medicine*, vol. 19, 7: 663–70.
38 Graham, H. (1984). *Women, Health and the Family*. Brighton, Wheatsheaf.
39 Roman, E., Beral, V. and Inskip, H. (1985). 'Occupational mortality among women in England and Wales' *British Medical Journal 1985*, 291: 194–6.
40 Whitehead, M. (1987). *The Health Divide*. London, Health Education Council.
41 Waldron, I. (1976). 'Why do women live longer than men?' *Social Science and Medicine*, vol. 10: 349–62.
42 Haavio-Mannila, E. (1986). 'Inequalities in health and gender' *Social Science and Medicine*, vol. 22 (2): 141–9.
43 Office of Populations, Censuses and Surveys (1988). op. cit.
44 Office of Populations, Censuses and Surveys (1986). op. cit.
45 Smith, A. and Jacobson, B. (1988). op. cit.
46 McClure, G. (1987). 'Suicide in England and Wales 1975–1984' *British Journal of Psychiatry*, 150: 309–14.
47 Goldberg, D. and Auxley, P. (1980). *Mental Illness in the Community*. London, Tavistock.
48 Blaxter, M. (1990). op. cit.
49 Blaxter, M. (1990). op. cit.
50 Wilkinson, R. (1986). 'Income and mortality', in Wilkinson, R. (ed.) *Class and Health: Research and Longitudinal Data*. London, Tavistock.

51 Wilkinson, R. (1986). op. cit.

52 Wilkinson, R. (1986). op. cit.

53 Wilkinson, R. (1989). 'Class mortality differentials, income distribution and trends in poverty 1921–1981' *Journal of Social Policy*, vol. 18, 3: 307–35.

54 British Medical Association (1987). *Deprivation and Ill-Health*. London, British Medical Association.

55 Cole-Hamilton, I. (1988). *Review of Food Patterns Amongst Lower Income Groups in the UK*, a Report to the Health Education Authority (unpublished).

56 Platt, S., Martin, C., Hunt, J. *et al.* (1989). 'Damp housing, mould growth and symptomatic health state' *British Medical Journal*, vol. 298: 1673–8.

57 Fisher, S. (1984). *Stress and Perceptions of Control*. London, Lawrence Erlbaum Associates.

58 Cole-Hamilton, I. (1988). op. cit.

59 Lang, T., Andrews, C., Hunt, J. *et al.* (1984). *Jam Tomorrow?* Food Policy Unit, Hollings Faculty, Manchester Polytechnic.

60 Cole-Hamilton, I. (1988). op. cit.

61 Wilkinson, R. (1989). op. cit.

3 | FOOD AND POVERTY

INTRODUCTION

Food plays a particularly important role in health throughout the life-course. Good health is dependent on not only having enough to eat, but also on eating a balanced amount of nutrients. In Britain in the 1920s and 1930s, the problems of food shortages and undernourishment due to poverty were major issues for social policy. Today, concern appears to revolve around the problems of dietary imbalances and over-consumption and their relationship to the so-called 'diseases of affluence'. As a result, food consumption is no longer seen as an issue for mainstream social policy, but rather the concern of health educators. Yet undernourishment due to poverty is still with us, raising the issue that lack of money for food is still a present-day social issue. This chapter aims to highlight the importance of food for the wider constituency of health and welfare workers, and not just those whose work is focused on health promotion.

The research suggests that poor families generally have unhealthier diets than their better-off counterparts. The poor have been chastised by politicians, the rich and health educators alike for their unhealthy diets and urged to opt for healthier eating patterns. Renewed interest in the relationship between the so-called 'diseases of affluence' and nutrition has heightened concern about eating patterns and led to a proliferation of new food and nutrition policies at both local and national level. These policies focus primarily on the role of individuals and their responsibility to choose healthy eating patterns. They rest on the assumption that our food choices are within our personal control. Within this context of individual responsibility for health, the poor diet of low-income families is often attributed to three main factors:

- inefficient food purchasing and irresponsible budgeting.
- preference for unhealthy foods.
- lack of knowledge concerning the value and composition of a healthy diet.

The idea that food choices and eating patterns rest on individual behaviour or knowledge dominates many health-education programmes and is the basis of much health and welfare work with families. Families are often given information about what constitutes a healthy diet or healthier cooking methods, 'encouraged' to spend their money more wisely and buy healthier food for the family diet. Yet our eating patterns are not only chosen, they are also constrained.

This chapter will examine the key questions 'Do low-income families eat a less healthy diet than their better-off counterparts, and if so why?' To attempt to answer these questions, and examine the validity of the 'ignorance and irresponsibility' explanations, this chapter will look at the following areas:

- *Patterns of food consumption and expenditure between families:* examining how patterns differ according to income and family structure.
- *Factors that influence family food choices:* focusing on the impact of household income, knowledge and attitudes to food, the cost of a healthy diet and the availability of healthy food.
- *Patterns of food intake within the family:* according to age, gender and type of household.
- *The effect of food poverty on health.*

FOOD PATTERNS BETWEEN FAMILIES

DO LOW-INCOME FAMILIES HAVE POORER DIETS? — PATTERNS OF FOOD INTAKE

A number of surveys have shown that families on low income are less likely to eat a healthy diet than families with high incomes.[1,2] These surveys have shown that low-income families are likely to eat less fresh fruit and vegetables, less fresh meat or fish, but more fatty foods, carbohydrate and filler foods, particularly sugar, white bread, jam, cakes and biscuits than high-income families. Table 3.1 summarizes the main differences in food intakes between high- and low-income families.

Patterns of food intake also vary according to family composition, as well as with household income. Data from the *Annual Report of the National Food Survey Committee (NFS)*, the main source of information on patterns of food consumption between households, suggests that average food consumption per person is higher in all-adult households, and lower in households with children. Average food consumption falls as numbers of children

TABLE 3.1   Food consumption by selected food items for high- and low-income families

Foods eaten more in low-income families	Foods eaten more in high-income families
White bread	Brown bread
Lard	Butter
Margarine	Cooking oils
Sugar	Cheese
Processed meats	Fresh carcass meat
Potatoes	Fruit
Canned vegetables	Fresh vegetables
Eggs	Poultry
Full-cream milk	Reduced-fat milk
Cereals	
Fish	
Preserves	

Source: Ministry of Agriculture, Food and Fisheries (1989). Household Food Consumption and Expenditure, Annual Report of the National Food Survey Committee, 1987. London, HMSO

increase.[3] Although this pattern generally remains the same across income groups, any reduction in individual consumption is most significant for low-income families, as their generally lower intake of food is compounded even further by the presence of children (see table 3.2). For example, a low-income family with two adults and three children has an average meat consumption that is only half the consumption of an equivalent-size, high-income family, and three times less than that of a low-income family that contains adults only. Although the presence of children appears to have an impact on food consumption patterns in families, there do not appear to be any differences between one- and two-parent households. Possible explanations for this will be considered later in this chapter, when food consumption patterns within families are discussed.

A lower consumption of food in low-income families with children implies that there will be a corresponding lower dietary intake of essential nutrients, unless low-income families are compensating in some way. However, as figure 3.1 (on page 56) indicates, low-income families are less likely to consume foods that are rich in essential nutrients, such as vitamins and minerals, or have a diet that is low in fats and sugar and high in dietary fibre, as recommended by the two major nutrition reports of the decade, the NACNE (National Advisory Committee on Nutrition Education) Report[4] and the COMA (Committee on Medical Aspects of Diet, Diet and Cardio-vascular Disease) Reports.[5] Although the NFS measures only the intake of selected nutrients, it shows lower intakes in low-income families than high-income families for nearly all the nutrients it records, particularly vitamin C. Yet, when the nutrient intake of vitamins is calculated as a

TABLE 3.2 Food consumption according to household composition with income groups, for selected food items (ounces per person per week)

	Highest-income group		Lowest-income group	
	Adults only	2 adults +3 children	Adults only	2 adults +3 children
Milk and creams (pints)	3.93	3.79	4.5	3.31
Cheese	6.04	4.37	4.69	2.19
Carcass meat	15.74	8.38	15.94	5.31
Other meat and meat products	22.82	17.56	28.55	19.34
Fish	7.51	5.10	6.66	2.14
Eggs (nos.)	3.12	1.95	3.73	2.88
Fats	10.39	6.88	12.95	8.07
Sugars and preserves	10.54	8.57	13.53	7.13
Potatoes	29.55	27.00	47.30	42.33
Fresh vegetables	41.04	24.3	35.12	15.30
Processed vegetables	16.53	14.75	19.10	17.35
Fresh fruit	33.14	22.04	21.41	7.80
Other fruit	16.14	17.81	10.22	3.68
Bread	28.32	23.80	36.28	30.23
Other cereals	23.49	25.97	26.49	20.29
Non-alcoholic drink	3.62	1.37	3.90	1.35
Total expenditure (per person)	£13.42	£9.39	£11.58	£5.61

Source: Ministry of Agriculture, Food and Fisheries (1989). Household Food Consumption and Expenditure, Annual Report of the National Food Survey Committee, 1987, London, HMSO

percentage of the recommended daily allowance in the NFS, it appears to be adequate for low-income families, with the exception of the intake of vitamin C. This could possibly be explained by the fact that the NFS records higher food intakes per person than weighed food surveys. Whilst weighed surveys take account only of food that is actually consumed, the NFS calculations are based on the amount of food brought into the house per week, regardless of whether it is consumed or not. Moreover, it does not take into account food that is consumed outside the home. As food consumption outside the home is increasing, particularly for high-income households, it is likely that if food consumed outside the home was taken into account, the NFS would show even greater differences in nutrient intakes between high- and low-income groups.

It is also worth noting that recommended daily allowances are thought to represent the amount of each nutrient required to prevent deficiency problems rather than the amounts required for optimum health. Moreover, the UK has lower recommended daily amounts for most nutrients than the United States or Europe.

MAJOR INFLUENCES ON FOOD CHOICES

In order to answer the question 'Why do low-income families eat a poorer diet than their better off counterparts?' it is useful to examine in more detail the effect that four factors have on food consumption and expenditure patterns: household income, knowledge and attitudes to food, the cost of a healthy diet and the availability of food. The next four sub-sections will examine each of these factors in turn.

HOUSEHOLD INCOME AND FOOD EXPENDITURE

Patterns of food consumption are closely linked to income and food expenditure. Food is the largest, single item of expenditure for most families. On average, approximately 19.6 per cent of the total household budget is spent on food.[6] However, the proportion of the budget and the amount spent on food varies between families according to household income, family composition and other competing costs, such as housing and fuel costs.

Low-income families spend a higher proportion of their total income on food than high-income families, leaving less money to spend on other health resources and luxury items (see figure 3.1).

Low-income families spend less in money terms, than families with higher incomes. Figure 3.1 shows the total weekly expenditure per household in low- and high-income families.

Low-income families also spend a larger proportion of their food budget on the types of food recommended by the various food policies as constituting a healthy diet. Although high-income groups spent more on healthy food than low-income groups in absolute terms in 1987, low-income families spent more of their income on healthy foods in relative terms. Data from the Family Expenditure Survey indicates that, in 1986, low-income families spent 60 per cent of their food budget on healthy foods, compared to high-income families who spent only 40 per cent on their food budget on healthy foods.[7]

Low-income families shop more efficiently in money and nutrient terms than higher-income families. Evidence that low-income families do not spend their food budget unwisely can be found in the NFS. In 1987 low-income families shopped more efficiently, buying nearly every type of food more cheaply than the national average price.[8] In addition to buying food more cheaply than high-income families, low-income families also buy food more efficiently in terms of nutritional content. Table 3.3 shows how low-income families bought approximately 25 per cent more of every nutrient, per £1 spent on food, than high-income families, with the exception of vitamin C.

So far the evidence does not support the view that inefficient food purchasing or irresponsible budgeting is responsible for the unhealthier diets of low-income families. To identify other possible explanations for

FIGURE 3.1   Proportion and amount of household expenditure spent on food (weekly) by income group (two-adult, two-children households)

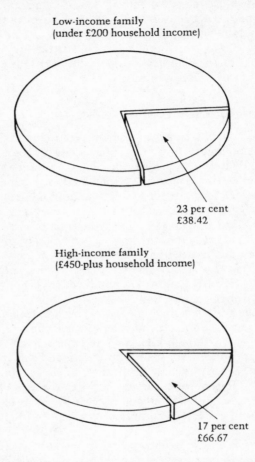

Low-income family
(under £200 household income)

23 per cent
£38.42

High-income family
(£450-plus household income)

17 per cent
£66.67

Source: Department of Employment (1990). *Family Expenditure Survey, 1988*. London, HMSO.

their poorer diets, it is necessary to turn now to examine whether unhealthy eating patterns amongst low-income families can be explained in terms of poor knowledge about the value and content of a healthy diet.

KNOWLEDGE AND ATTITUDES TO FOOD

Underlying much current health-education advice and literature is an assumption that many people do not change to healthier eating patterns because they lack information about the value and composition of a healthy

TABLE 3.3   Amount of nutrients bought per £1 spent on food for high- and low-income households, 1987

	High-income household	Low-income household		Difference between high- and low-income households %
		With earner	Without earner	
Energy(KCal)	170.3	230	221	35
Protein(g)	5.8	7.6	7.2	31
Fat(g)	7.9	10.72	10.2	35
Carbohydrate(g)	20.2	27.7	26.7	38
Calcium(g)	75	98	93	30
Iron(mg)	0.97	1.2	1.2	24
Thiamine(mg)	0.11	0.15	0.14	36
Riboflavin(mg)	0.15	0.19	0.18	27
Niacin(mg)	2.4	3.0	2.8	25
Vitamin C(mg)	6.6	5.6	5.6	15
Vitamin A(mg)	98.6	143	142	45
Vitamin D(mg)	0.26	0.34	0.35	31
Amount spent (weekly)	£11.86	£8.58	£9.71	

Source: Calculated from Ministry of Agriculture, Food and Fisheries (1989). *Household Food Consumption and Expenditure, Annual Report of the National Food Survey Committee, 1987*. London, HMSO

diet. In particular, the diets of poor families and Black and ethnic-minority families have been identified as the result of ignorance and singled out as a target for change. In the last decade a number of studies have examined people's knowledge about the value and composition of a healthy diet. The results of these studies indicate that, contrary to many assumptions, low-income groups have fairly good knowledge about the value and composition of a healthy diet, and similar levels of knowledge to high income groups.

Lang *et al.*'s study (1984) of low-income groups in the north of England found that 85 per cent of respondents thought diet was important for health and showed considerable concern about the health effects of too much fat, sugar, additives and colourings.[9]

Calnan's study (1988) found that women in social classes I and II and social classes IV and V mentioned diet, along with exercise, most frequently as important for health. Women in both the top and bottom social classes both had a good awareness of the composition of a healthy diet.[10]

Data from the NFS suggests that both high- and low-income groups have been changing their eating patterns along the lines of current nutritional advice, since the early 1980s. In both income groups consumption of wholemeal bread and potatoes has increased, and consumption of fat, sugar, biscuits and cakes has declined. However, while fruit and vegetable consumption has increased marginally in the higher-income groups, consumption has actually declined in low-income groups. This may be associated with the fact that fruit and vegetable prices have increased significantly in comparison to many other foods since 1982. In view of changing eating patterns in both high- and low-income groups, there are signs that, within the limits of their income, the poorest groups may have responded to nutritional advice to the same extent as other groups.[11] In this light we can see that unhealthy eating patterns are not simply a matter of ignorance or a careless attitude towards health. Even when knowledge about and attitudes towards healthy eating are positive, other factors, such as the cost and availability of food, may override our feelings and influence our eating and expenditure patterns.

COST OF A HEALTHY DIET

A commonly held assumption is that a healthy diet does not necessarily cost more than an unhealthy diet. However, this assumption does not seem to fit in with the facts. People can eat only the food they can afford to buy. Families with low incomes need to economize to keep their food costs down, as well as maximizing the amount of calories and nutrients they get for their money. The foods eaten more frequently by low-income families tend to cost less than those eaten by higher-income households. Invariably cheaper food has high fat or sugar contents or low fibre contents. For example, fatty minced beef is far cheaper than lean mince beef, and white bread is considerably cheaper than wholemeal bread but has less fibre. Moreover, healthy foods appear to have undergone greater price increases than less healthy foods (see table 3.4).

Although many 'healthier' alternatives to cheaper food are lower in fat and sugar and higher in fibre, they also contain fewer calories, which must then be made up from other foods. This may have the effect of increasing the food bill even further. This may have little effect on high-income families

TABLE 3.4 Increases in food prices, 1982–6

Healthy foods	%	Less healthy foods	%
Wholemeal bread	17	White bread	15
Green vegetables	17–51	Biscuits	19
Root vegetables	29–37	Sugar	13
Salad vegetables	22–42	Bacon	13
Fresh fruit	16–45	Sausages	13
Poultry	26	Whole milk	17
Fish	44	Butter	9

Source: Health Visitor Journal, December 1989, vol. 62, no. 12

but is likely to be beyond the means of low-income families. Cole-Hamilton[12] has calculated that a simple piece of dietary advice such as 'throw away the frying pan' is likely to increase the cost of the family food bill. Cooking fats, despite the fact that they may raise the level of fat in the blood and increase the risk of coronary heart disease, provide a valuable and cheap source of calories for low-income families. To replace these calories with alternatives which are more in line with dietary advice would have cost between 12p and £2.05 per week per person in 1986.

However, not all foods eaten by low-income families are cheap sources of calories or nutrients, for example, biscuits and cakes. Although low-income families spend a higher proportion of their food expenditure on biscuits and cakes, they actually spend far less in money terms than high-income families.[13] Low-income families could cut out biscuits and cakes or eat cheaper and healthier alternatives to meat products, such as beans and pulses. However, food such as beans and pulses can have higher cooking costs, due to the longer time they take to cook, in comparison to many other foods. Moreover, eating is a social activity as well as a health activity. It may well be unrealistic to expect certain groups to make food choices that are not in line with commonly accepted eating patterns, or to deny themselves any pleasure from eating. What is commonly accepted and familiar food is not just a matter of personal taste, but a matter of previous experience, and hence food traditions. The social importance of food will be discussed later in this chapter.

Several attempts have been made in recent years, to compare the approximate costs of 'healthy' and 'unhealthy' diets. Shopping basket surveys carried out in various parts of the country indicate that a healthy diet can cost up to 35 per cent more than an unhealthy diet.[14] Cole-Hamilton,[15] commenting on the evidence collected over the last four years suggests:

> the cost of a diet in line with current dietary advice, which takes into account individual preferences and social factors, costs significantly more than the amount most people with low incomes in the UK are able to spend.

Several attempts have been made to calculate whether families on low income can afford to buy healthy foods. The Maternity Alliance[16] has estimated that the cost of an adequate diet for an expectant mother may be beyond the means of families who are dependent on benefits or low wages. These mothers may have to spend up to half of their income on food if they conform to the dietary advice given to them by maternity hospitals, leaving very little money to pay housing, fuel and other bills. The new age-related structure of income support means that young women, in particular, receive very low-scale rates, leaving very little money for food.

Research in progress at Brunel University indicates that social-security rates for children are totally inadequate for the nutritional needs of a growing child. The research indicates that, even if full claims are made for free school meals and free milk, the income-support-scale rates would only allow for 86 per cent of the nutritional needs of a 5-year-old and 68 per cent of the needs of an 8-year-old.[17]

Lang et al.'s[18] calculations suggest that families with people with special needs and disabilities may find it difficult to find the money to pay for special diets. Families with people with disabilities and special needs often have lower incomes and higher expenditure than other groups (see chapter 1), increasing the pressure on food resources. The additional costs of special diets may be beyond the budgets of low-income families with people with special needs. Lang et al. calculated that a high-fibre diet recommended by a family doctor cost £16.86 per week in November, 1985. This would have accounted for 57 per cent of the total income for a single householder receiving supplementary benefit at 1985 scale rates but would have been partly off-set by a special diet addition of £11.30 per week (which is no longer available under the new income-support scheme).

For many low-income families a healthy diet may cost more than their budget allows, forcing them to buy cheaper foods, despite the higher fat and sugar and lower fibre contents. The daily food hardships and struggles of low-income families are reflected in a number of studies that have looked at food poverty and the realities of breadline living. These studies indicate that some low-income families have to cut back on food expenditure and consumption when money is short.[19,20,21] Unlike housing costs, fuel bills or debt payments, food is a flexible item in the family budget on which expenditure can be decreased or increased, depending on the amount of money available each week. Although food expenditure may be cut when money is short, it is still seen as the most important priority of household expenditure by the majority of low-income families.[22]

> Food is the only place I find I can tighten up. The rest of it, they take it before you get your hands on it really. So it's the food . . . The only thing I can cut down on is food . . .
>
> (Lone mother with two children)[23]

Whilst surveys of family food circumstances indicate that low-income families may not have enough money to buy healthy foods, they draw our attention to another important fact: *families in poverty may not even have enough money to feed every member of the family at each meal, each day.*

 Lang's et al.'s study of food hardship in the north of England indicated that 25 per cent of respondents had missed a meal in the last year because of money difficulties. Twelve per cent of respondents said they did not have enough money for food all week, and 38 per cent had only just enough money for food all week.[24]

 Burghes's study of families on supplementary benefit showed that 15 per cent of children and 75 per cent of adults had fewer than three meals a day when money was short.[25]

Whilst all families with low incomes are likely to struggle to find enough money to provide themselves with enough food and a healthy diet, families with children appear to experience particular food hardships. The health and nutritional problems they experience will be discussed later in this chapter.[26]

FOOD AVAILABILITY

For people to eat in line with current dietary advice, healthy foods must be readily available to buy. Surveys that have looked at food availability indicate that healthy foods are often less readily available than unhealthy foods.[27] These shopping surveys have concentrated on towns and cities and have indicated that less prosperous localities have the most limited access to healthy foods. Changes in the food retailing market have seen a decline in the local shop as more supermarkets have been built on the outskirts of towns and cities. As a consequence, less food is available to buy at local level. Whilst this causes problems for people in towns or cities, the problems may be even greater for rural people who may have to travel great distances to find a good selection of healthy foods. Where local shops do exist, they often have poor stocks of fresh foods, particularly fruit and vegetables, as shopkeepers find it easier to stock and sell foods that are less perishable.

Food also tends to be more expensive at shops with limited food stocks. A survey by the London Food Commission (1985)[28] found that low-income families in London had to pay around £4.50 more per week if they shopped in a store that had a reduced range of food items. Although local shops tend to be expensive, the fact that they will often split packs of food, such as eggs and fruit (and nappies and cigarettes), and sell items singly, makes them attractive to shoppers with limited budgets. Although large supermarkets stock a large variety of healthy foods, shopping at supermarkets frequently involves travelling some distance. This adds to the cost of food, as well as being difficult for families without cars, and groups such as people with disabilities, older adults and mothers with young children.

Unfortunately, the NFS does not give us any information about the consumption and expenditure patterns of minority ethnic families. Yet food availability is frequently a problem for Black and minority ethnic families. Many traditional foods are not readily available and families may have to travel considerable distances to buy food. As many foods have been imported, they tend to cost more than many foods used in the British diet. Although many areas with a large number of minority ethnic families now have shops that specialize in traditional foods, some families still live in areas away from other members of their own culture. Where traditional foods are less available, families may be forced to buy traditional British foods without information about the nutrient content or health value of these foods or to rely on a restricted range of their own traditional foods.

The National Food Survey is an invaluable source of data on food-consumption patterns between low- and high-income families. It draws our attention to the food hardships of low-income families who, despite efficient food budgeting and management strategies, are often unable to afford the cost of a healthy diet and, in some circumstances, not even the cost of three meals a day for all the family. Low pay, inadequate social-security benefits and the relatively high cost of healthy foods compromises both the quality and quantity of foods consumed by low-income families.

FOOD DISTRIBUTION WITHIN FAMILIES

The NFS gives us a useful insight into the distribution of food resources between families. However, it obscures food consumption patterns within families. Food is a health resource that is not shared equally by all members of the family. Men, women and children eat differently in terms of quality and quantity. Whilst a family's access to food is determined by the forces we discussed in the first part of this chapter, that is, income, food attitudes and knowledge, and food availability and costs, food consumption patterns within the family are influenced by another set of factors. The distribution of food within families appears to be closely related to age, gender and family structure. Research has shown that factors such as the social signifi-cance of food, food preferences, the role food plays in behaviour manage-ment and money management patterns within the family mediate an individual's access to food along gender and age lines. As a result, some members of a family may find their food intake, and hence nutritional state, compromised by social relationships within the home. Patterns of food distribution within the home illustrate the complex division of responsi-bilities and resources within the family[29] and mark out the roles of men and women and of parents and children. The next five sub-sections will exam-ine, in turn, food patterns within families, the social significance of food, food preferences, food in behaviour control and money management pat-terns. The majority of the data in these sub-sections refers to white families only. In the absence of research data on Black and minority ethnic groups it is easy to fall into the trap of making assumptions based on stereotypical ideas about eating habits in families. It is important to acknowledge that food consumption patterns differ between and within Black and minority ethnic families, just as they do in white families.

FOOD CONSUMPTION PATTERNS WITHIN THE FAMILY

Food consumption patterns within the family are strongly related to age and gender. Several studies have indicated how eating patterns differ between white men and women. Men eat more food than women.[30] Men eat 'proper' meals (carcass meat and two vegetables) more frequently than women.[31,32] Women tend to eat more brown bread, fruit and salad than men.[33] Eating patterns also differ according to age. Children eat more cereal, milk, sweets and biscuits than their parents,[34] and more convenience foods; fish fingers, burgers, beans.[35] Children are also less likely than their parents to miss meals when money is short.[36] To understand why eating patterns differ within families we need to examine the social significance of food within the home.

THE SOCIAL SIGNIFICANCE OF FOOD WITHIN THE FAMILY

Research into the food circumstances of families confirms that food management is still women's work in the majority of homes.[37] The provision of meals for the family is a responsibility that women, as carers, take very seriously. Being a mother involves managing the household budget at the same time as managing the responsibility for the family's health. Families are often judged by the quality of their food. A good home is where the children are well fed, and a good mother is seen as someone who provides nourishing food for her family.

Several studies of white, British families have shown that women attach both social, as well as nutritional significance to the provision of a 'proper' meal.[38,39] For many women, a 'proper' meal is a cooked dinner which consists of carcass meat with two fresh vegetables and should be consumed on a daily basis. The typical British Sunday dinner epitomizes a 'proper' meal. Cheaper alternatives, such as beefburgers, fish fingers, chips and baked beans, are seen as lower status food and are rarely seen to constitute a 'proper' meal. The relatively high cost of a 'proper' meal, particularly carcass meat, means that when money for food is short, women may have either to cut down on the number of 'proper' meals they are able to provide or to cut down on other areas of food consumption. The relatively high cost of high-status food may mean that a 'proper' meal is beyond the means of a low-income family altogether, forcing them to consume less healthy alternatives. Low-income families may be very reluctant to change their eating patterns radically to consume the cheaper and healthier alternatives recommended by some health-education programmes, such as pulses and beans, or vegetarian food because they lack the social significance of more familiar foods.

Some research studies suggests that certain gender differences in food consumption, particularly the consumption of meat, may be explained in terms of the relative status and power of different family members.[40] Charles and Kerr[41] suggest that high-status foods and proper meals are more frequently associated with men than women and reflect their high status as breadwinner in the household. While historically and in many present-day cultures food is an indicator of social worth, and the best food is served to the most prestigious person, it is unlikely that differences in meat consumption among white families of British origin can be explained solely in terms of status and power. Differences in meat consumption between men and women are now small.[42] Women generally have healthier diets, consuming slightly less red meat, less fatty food and sugar and more fruit, vegetables and salad. The food industry targets many 'healthy' foods at women, whilst less healthy foods such as red meat and alcohol are promoted as masculine foods. In addition to targeting certain foods at men and women, the food industry also markets certain foods as children's foods. The higher consumption of lower-status foods, such as fish fingers, and beefburgers, may be due to marketing and the kind of food preferences children develop as much as to children's status within the home.

Moreover, gender differences in food consumption do not necessarily reflect differences in living standards between men and women. Pahl's latest research suggests that in many households men and women share a common standard of living, although there is a substantial minority of households where the male partner has a more affluent standard of living than his female partner.[43] Differences in living standards relating to food will be discussed later in this chapter.

Whilst we have a wealth of information about the social significance of certain foods for white families of British origin, we have very little research data on the way the social significance of food influences food distribution within Black and minority ethnic families. However, we do know that Black and minority ethnic families are at greater risk of poverty than many white families. As a result, they may have difficulty in conforming to culturally and socially acceptable eating patterns. For some members of Black and minority ethnic groups food has a religious significance. Food patterns between and within families may reflect the religious significance of food. Religious food restrictions differ within individual minority groups depending on individual views. Again, we need to remember that stereotypical ideas about the religious significance of food in families often bear little resemblance to the food patterns of Black and minority ethnic groups.

FOOD PREFERENCES

The food preferences of adults and children also shape family eating patterns. In some two-parent families, the tastes and preferences of the male partner may determine the content of the main meal of the day. Charles and Kerr's[44] study of attitudes towards feeding and nutrition in young children indicated that the male partner's preferences and the female partner's feeling that men deserve a 'proper' meal tended to make the main meal of the day more traditional and elaborate and, hence, more expensive, than other meals. The accounts of food consumption in lone-parent families suggest that meals are likely to be less traditional and elaborate when there is no male partner's preferences to take into account.[45]

Children's food preferences also help to shape family eating patterns. Although children appear to have less direct control over the content of their diet than the male head of household, children's food preferences appear to have an indirect effect on the family diet: children may not always be allowed to choose what they want to eat, but mothers frequently select food they know their children prefer.[46] Charles and Kerr[47] suggest that children's food preferences may be most influential when there is no male adult present to subordinate their food preferences, for example, when father is absent or in lone-mother families. Providing food is an integral part of loving and caring for a child. By selecting food they know their children will like, parents not only get the pleasure of seeing their children eat, but they also minimize the risk of the foods being wasted. Often children's food preferences do not fall into line with current dietary advice. Foods that are usually palatable to young children – fish fingers, beefburgers, beans and flavoured yoghurts – are often foods that are high in fat and sugar and low in fibre.

Low-income families cannot afford to offer foods that are likely to be wasted. This may lead to a reluctance to accept healthy-eating advice that suggests the introduction of new foods into the family diet. Food preferences may be a stronger determinant of eating patterns than health-education advice when money is short. For many families it is better to fill up on something, even if it is less healthy, than risk refusal when an alternative is difficult to provide.

> I usually cook . . . sort of really more for what they like so that I don't have anything to throw away. Like I know they wouldn't eat either liver or kidneys so I just never buy it you see, I cook and buy things I know they'll eat . . .
>
> (Woman whose husband is unemployed)[48]

FOOD AND BEHAVIOUR CONTROL

As well as being a way of expressing love, food can also be used to control behaviour and avoid conflict. Mealtimes are a time for socializing children to eat at a socially accepted time and in a socially accepted way. As a result, mealtimes are often a time of conflict, as children use the opportunity to rebel against parental authority and assert their own will by refusing to eat. By offering food they know their children will eat, parents are often able to avoid stress and conflict at mealtimes. For low-income families worries about food are likely to compound the general stress of poverty. Giving way to children's food preferences may be one way that poor parents cope with the stress of life on or below the breadline.

Parents use food to control their children and also to punish and reward them. For example, sweets and biscuits may be used to keep a tired and irritable child quiet during shopping trips or when preparing food. Whilst many health and welfare workers often discourage parents from using sweets and biscuits as treats, or as a way of controlling children's behaviour, they are cheaper, more convenient and less messy alternatives to other healthier foods, such as fresh fruit. Although sweets and biscuits are of little nutritional value, and indeed can be health damaging, paradoxically they act as an important health resource for many families. Parents appear to use these foods to help them reconcile their childcare responsibilities with other caring and household responsibilities (see chapter 6). Other feeding decisions also appear to fall into this pattern. Early introduction of solids or adding baby cereal to baby milk may be a way of coping with a crying or restless baby. Changing from breast to bottle feeding may be the easiest way a mother can find time for herself and other family members. Food decisions that may appear irrational or irresponsible to health and welfare workers may be a rational way of coping with stressful situations in low-income families.

FAMILY FOOD DISTRIBUTION AND MONEY MANAGEMENT

Women's accounts of factors that affect their ability to care for family health have highlighted that money arrangements within the home shape both patterns of caring and the standard of living of each individual family member, including access to food. Studies of financial arrangements within families have usually concentrated on arrangements within marriage or marriage-type relationships. They have highlighted that, whilst a variety of systems exist for organizing money within families, crucial to them all are the issues of who *controls* money within the home and who *manages* the budget on a day-to-day basis. Couples often separate the control and management of money along gender lines, with control and key decisions about how money will be allocated resting with male partners, while day-to-day management of allocated expenditure rests with the female partner.[49] Wilson's survey of financial arrangements within marriage-type relationships indicated that male control over expenditure may increase as income rises. In low-income households women were usually completely responsible for all expenditure and coped reasonably well within the limits of the income, as long as their partners did not keep too much money for themselves. As women lost control over expenditure, the hardship for them and their children increased. As income levels rose, male partners became increasingly involved in the payment of bills and food expenditure. Although money problems arise far less often, women in high-income homes may not necessarily have an opportunity to implement their own spending priorities unless they have incomes of their own.[50]

For women with poor access to household income, independent sources of income, however small, become very significant. Child benefit is the main source of independent income available to mothers. It appears to act as a vital safety net for women. First, it is paid directly to mothers, bypassing male control. Second, it has an important role in budgeting. Many women who receive child benefit on a weekly basis use it to pay for school meals or supplement the food budget, whilst those who receive it monthly often use it to pay for more major items of expenditure, such as bills and clothing.[51] Unfortunately the gradual erosion of the monetary value of child benefit means that women are less able to use it as a safety net.

The controlling influence of a male partner on a mother's access to money may bring women's responsibilities for caring for family health into conflict with her responsibilities for managing the household budget, particularly keeping the family out of debt. As we identified earlier, food costs are often met after fixed costs, such as housing and fuel bills, have been paid. Thus food is often purchased when the household budget is most depleted. When money for health resources is short, either because of low family income, or because a woman's access to the household income is restricted by her partner, women as managers of family resources are faced with the task of containing family poverty. Surveys of how women cope with poverty indicate that they often seek to do this by, first, cutting their personal expenditure, and second, when this cannot be cut any further, they cut their personal consumption. Commonly they cut their own consumption of food to reduce the effects of food hardship on the rest of the family.[52,53] This research indicates that women at all income levels make personal food sacrifices when necessary. This suggests that even at high income levels women may experience food poverty and inadequate nutrient intake. However, women in low-income families are most likely to have to make cuts in their own food consumption. The research indicates that personal food sacrifices are commonest amongst lone mothers. The overall poverty of lone parents forces them to take steps to reduce expenditure and consumption to a greater extent than two-parent families. In Graham's study (1987)[54] of mothers with pre-school children, 68 per cent of lone mothers and 35 per cent of mothers in two-parent families identified their diets as an area for cutbacks.

Although many lone mothers are likely to have less household income than women with partners, they are no longer subject to the spending priorities of partners. As a consequence, some lone mothers find it easier to cut back on personal food consumption than mothers in two-parent families. In lone-parent households the distinction between control and management of money and resources is dissolved, giving women the power to organize and spend their money as they wish. For these reasons, many lone mothers can feel financially better off outside marriage, despite the fact that they may have reduced incomes and increased costs, such as those for childcare. This may explain why lone-parent families do not have different food consumption patterns from other two-parent families. Whilst many lone parents have the power to improve the family diet, paradoxically they may use this power to make greater cutbacks in their own food consumption. In dietary terms, the personal health costs may be great. While we have no evidence of the nutritional content of the diets of lone mothers, lone mothers themselves are more likely than women in two-parent families to rate their own diet as poor.[55] 'I'm better-off I think. Although I have less money, it's all mine to allocate where I want . . . It's harder to make ends meet but I know where the money is so it's easier for me' (a lone mother with two children).[56]

THE EFFECT OF FOOD POVERTY ON HEALTH

The relationship between food poverty and ill health is now well known. Whilst the poor health status of low-income families is due to the effects of multiple disadvantage, it is clear that the quality and quantity of the food they eat have an adverse effect on their health. Although all low-income families are likely to find it difficult to consume a healthy diet, certain groups appear to experience particular food hardships and have an increased risk of nutritional deprivation due to low income. The next six sub-sections will consider the effects of nutritional deprivation on children, parents, pregnant women, Black and minority ethnic families, homeless families and families with people with special needs.

CHILDREN

The additional costs of children are not adequately compensated for by state benefits. Child benefit, the only source of additional income available universally to mothers, has been frozen since 1988 and has not increased in line with inflation since 1985. School meals can no longer be relied on to provide a nutritious meal for poor children. Research in the 1970s and early 1980s, when free school meals were more widely available and provided at low cost for other children, has indicated that school meals can be a major source of energy and nutrients for children from low-income families.[57] Since 1980 local education authorities are no longer obliged to provide nutritionally balanced meals or meals at low cost. The nutritional standard of meals is thought to have deteriorated in many schools, particularly as some local education authorities now provide only a sandwich lunch for children entitled to free school meals. While children from families on income support are still entitled to free school meals, children from families on family credit and other low-income families lost their entitlement under the Social Security Act, 1986. Whilst children usually fare better than their parents in terms of meals, there is strong evidence to suggest that their diet is compromised by poverty. Many children are deprived of healthy food through lack of income at a time when their need for nutrients is at its greatest. Poor diet in childhood is associated with a variety of problems, including poor physical and intellectual growth and development, obesity, dental caries and diseases associated with vitamin and mineral deficiencies, such as anaemia and rickets. Moreover, there is a growing body of evidence that suggests that the major public health problems of the decade, in particular, coronary heart disease, have their origins in childhood.

A study of children from deprived socio-economic groups showed that they are often smaller in stature than their peers.[58]

 Dental caries are commonest in children from the most socially and economically deprived homes.[59]

 Iron, calcium, and protein intakes can be very low for children from socially and economically deprived homes.[60]

A survey of the diets of British school children showed that the majority of children from all social groups had diets that were too high in fat and low in fibre. Girls also had low levels of iron and calcium.[61]

PARENTS

As we have seen, parents frequently mitigate the effects of food poverty on their children by cutting down on their own food consumption. Mothers also appear to experience high levels of stress at meal-times which, for some women, distracts them from eating their own food. Mothers are particularly vulnerable to food poverty. Not only are they more likely than their partners to sacrifice their own food for other family members, and to be wholly dependent on food produced at home, but they are also more likely to be earning wages that are below the poverty line. This has particular consequences for lone mothers and their children. Young parents are likely to be especially at risk of nutritional deprivation and food poverty. The age-related structure of income support means that young parents receive very low-scale rates for themselves. Nutritional deficiencies during childbearing years not only have consequences for the health of parents, they also affect the health of unborn children. The nutritional state of the parents before conception, as well as during pregnancy, is thought to affect the health of the child. Not only do parents go without food when money is short, the evidence suggests that they also have diets that are too high in fat and sugar and too low in fibre. Higher rates of coronary heart disease and bowel cancer among poorer social classes may be partly explained by the high-fat and low-fibre content of the diets of adults living in poverty.

 In a survey of people aged 15–25 years, men with low incomes had the lowest average intakes of thiamin, vitamin C and calcium and women had the lowest average intakes of protein, calcium, thiamine and riboflavin.[62]

PREGNANT WOMEN

The importance of diet in pregnancy is well established. Poor diet in pregnancy has been shown to be associated with low birth weight, perinatal death and some congenital malformations, such as spina bifida. As the nutritional state of the mother is likely to improve with income, nutritional differences in pregnancy may partly explain why babies born to mothers in lower social classes have lower birth weights and higher perinatal death rates. The Maternity Alliance's analysis of the cost of an adequate diet for expectant mothers shows that some pregnant women on low incomes will face great difficulties in paying for a healthy diet which is in line with dietary advice.

 A survey of pregnant women on supplementary benefit showed that one-third of the pregnant women consumed a very poor diet.[63]

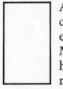 A survey of pregnant women in a socially and economically deprived area showed that some mothers from lower socio-economic groups had serious nutritional deficits in pregnancy. Mothers of infants with low birth weights (less than 2500 grams) had significantly lower intakes of energy during pregnancy than mothers of heavier babies.[64]

BLACK AND MINORITY ETHNIC FAMILIES

Although we have very little research on food patterns among Black and minority ethnic groups, in the light of what we know about their economic and social situations, it is likely that many families find it difficult to make healthy food choices within the limits of their income. Many traditional foods are not always readily available, and they may be more expensive than other foods. Low income and lack of access to reasonably priced traditional foods are rarely used to explain health choices and nutritional problems among Black and minority ethnic groups. Nutritional problems tend to be more readily explained in terms of the inherent deficiencies of Black and minority ethnic diets, with health education and more information, rather than food and income policies, seen as the solution to the problems. For example, a health-education campaign to reduce the incidence of rickets was chosen in preference to the fortification of chappati flour, even though rickets has only been eradicated from the white majority group with the fortification of margarine. Black and minority ethnic groups also have poorer access to useful dietary advice. Health-education messages are often based on the white, British diet and fail to incorporate foods and eating patterns that are familiar to individual Black and minority ethnic groups. Moreover, they also fail to provide information in different languages. Although high rates of some diseases, such as rickets and heart disease among some Black and minority ethnic groups have been blamed on diet, the extent to which these diseases have dietary causes is unclear.

The diets of Asian children have been found deficient in iron and vitamin D.[65]

FAMILIES WITH PEOPLE WITH SPECIAL NEEDS

As we saw in chapter 1, special needs and disability increase an individual's propensity towards poverty. Many special therapeutic diets cost significantly more than normal food, and more than the average person spends on food each week. Since the Social Security Act, 1986, the supplementary-benefit weekly additional payments for special requirements have been abolished, including additions for special diets. The Disability Alliance[66] has calculated that many people with disabilities may be receiving up to £50 per week less under the new income-support scheme. Some families with children with disabilities have been particularly hard hit. The disabled child's premium is only available to families who are entitled to claim attendance or mobility allowance, yet many children with severe disabilities are too young for this entitlement. Therefore the extra food and other costs must be met out of existing benefits or wages, regardless of how inadequate they are. The additional costs of getting to the shops to buy food for families with people with disabilities only adds to the costs of food. It appears that those with dietary needs over and above those of others are likely to suffer the worst food hardships.

HOMELESS FAMILIES

Not only are homeless families likely to have very poor access to cooking and food-storage facilities, they often have to subsidize accommodation costs with money from food allowances. Food allowances for homeless families are unlikely to cover the cost of food all week. This is particularly worrying as many homeless families are families with young children.

 In a survey by the London Borough of Camden, only 6 out of 299 hotels used for homeless people provided accommodation that was within the cash limits offered.[67]

 Two-thirds of health visitors who responded to a Health Visitor Association/Shelter survey indicated that malnutrition was a common problem for homeless families.[68]

 Weight loss is common among homeless adults, and low birth weight is common among babies born to mothers in temporary accommodation.[69]

CONCLUSION AND IMPLICATIONS FOR PRACTICE

The problem of food poverty remains a present-day social problem. The tendency for low-income families to have less healthy diets than their wealthier counterparts is often attributed by politicians, professionals and the general public alike to ignorance and irresponsible behaviour. These assumptions underlie not only nutrition policies, but health-education programmes. However, data from the National Food Survey and numerous surveys of food consumption and expenditure patterns inform us that we need to understand the eating patterns of low-income families in the light of information about the cost and availability of healthy food, and the role that food plays in family life. Low income, mediated by age and gender, appear to determine the eating patterns of poor families. Whilst knowledge and attitudes to food undoubtedly play a part, there is no evidence to suggest that low-income families are any more ignorant about the content or importance of a healthy diet than the rest of society in the UK.

The links between good health and food are well documented. Food affects health through physiological processes, determining the body's ability to grow and develop, and resist disease throughout the life-cycle. This chapter clearly illustrates that behavioural and psychological processes also play an important and often misunderstood role in the relationship between food and health. Material and social factors, such as low income, available shopping facilities, the cost of food, age, gender and our beliefs about the social significance of food influence our eating behaviour and, hence, our health. Our food choices, like other health choices, do not occur in a vacuum nor are they simply the result of our knowledge and attitudes to food. Food also affects our health through psychological processes. The stress, isolation and depression that result from low income, poor housing, homelessness and unemployment make food purchasing and preparation a demanding task. The additional stresses of coping with a young child in a restricting environment make healthy eating choices even more difficult.

This review of the relationship between food, poverty and health informs us that we need to develop a more dynamic approach towards family health-education programmes. Misconceptions about the factors that affect family food choices and lack of political will to acknowledge the links between the material conditions of people's lives and health have led to a situation where the bulk of preventive health policy and education programmes are targeted at individuals. Yet the information in this chapter alerts us to the fact that individual approaches to health education are unlikely to bring about the desired behaviour changes or reduce the diseases of the late nineteenth century until the factors that constrain food and other health choices are removed. First, household income is a key, if not sole, factor in improving the eating patterns of low-income families, and chapter 1 highlighted the need for social security, taxation, employment and wage policies that improve the material conditions and incomes of the poor. Second, there is a need for food production and marketing policies at national and international level that bring healthy eating choices within the reach of all families. Present-day policies mean that healthy alternatives are the most expensive and least available choices and often give us little option but to eat high-additive, processed food. Moreover, food policies have created food mountains while the poor of Britain and the rest of the world suffer food shortages.

The research that highlights the relationship between food, poverty and health leaves many health and welfare workers with a feeling of powerlessness, a feeling that many of the factors that shape food choices are out of their control. Yet as practitioners, health and welfare workers have the responsibility to help families mitigate and cope with the effects of poverty. The acknowledgement of the links between food poverty and health has led some workers to question the value of traditional approaches which aim to change individual behaviour and to turn to new approaches that recognize the material constraints of breadline living. Food co-operatives, free or cheap community-transport shopping schemes and the provision of community eating facilities, where healthy meals are available at low cost, are examples of initiatives that help families mitigate and cope with the effects of food poverty. Some workers have discovered that some families have found budget-cookery courses useful, although the same courses have also been used to reinforce the belief that poor families simply need to improve their knowledge of healthy food. It can also be argued that the relationship between food and poverty demands that practitioners use their knowledge about food poverty to give information that is useful to families with low incomes, unlike many health-education messages which are largely irrelevant as a guide for action.[70] Information on social-security benefits and using the social-security system, information and help to gain access to childcare facilities which enable women to get a break from their children, or information on other forms of social support in the community are areas of work that may be more appropriate to families in food poverty than 'throw out the chip pan' type advice. Moreover, knowledge about food poverty means that fieldworkers need to continue to improve their skills to work in partnership with parents and acknowledge that parents often have the knowledge to assess their own health needs. Finally, the need for workers to play a role in shaping and informing nutrition and social policies at local and national level, through information sharing, research and the use of professional organizations, emerges as an important and legitimate area of professional work.

REFERENCES

1 Milburn, J., Clarke, A. and Smith, F. (1987). *Nae Bread*. Health Education Department, Argyll and Clyde Health Board.
2 Lang, T., Andrews, C., Bedale, C. *et al.* (1984). *Jam Tomorrow?* Food Policy Unit, Hollings Faculty, Manchester Polytechnic.
3 Ministry of Agriculture, Fisheries and Food (1989). *Household Food Consumption and Expenditure. Annual Report of National Food Survey Committee.* London, HMSO.

4 Health Education Council (1983). National Advisory Committee on Nutrition Education, *Proposals for Nutritional Guide-lines in Britain: a Discussion Paper*. London, HMSO.
5 Department of Health and Social Security (1984). Committee on Medical Aspects of Diet, Diet and Cardiovascular Disease, *Report on Health and Social Subjects No. 28*. London, HMSO.
6 Department of Employment (1988). *Family Expenditure Survey*. London, HMSO.
7 Department of Employment (1988). op. cit.
8 Ministry of Agriculture, Fisheries and Food (1989). op. cit.
9 Lang, T. *et al*. (1984). op. cit.
10 Calnan, M. (1988). 'Food and health: a comparison of beliefs and practices in middle class and working class households', in Cunningham-Birley, S. and McKegary, N. (eds) *Readings in Medical Sociology*. London, Tavistock.
11 Whitehead, M. (1987). *The Health Divide: Inequalities in Health in the 1980's*. London, Health Education Council.
12 Cole-Hamilton, I. (1988). *Review of Food Patterns Amongst Lower Income Groups in the UK*, a Report to the Health Education Authority (unpublished).
13 Department of Employment (1988). op. cit.
14 Cole-Hamilton, I. (1988). op. cit.
15 Cole-Hamilton, I. (1988). op. cit.
16 Durward, L. (1988). *Poverty in Pregnancy: The Cost of An Adequate Diet for Expectant Mothers*. London, Maternity Alliance.
17 Brunel University *Research in Progress*. Cited by Cole-Hamilton, I. (1988). op. cit.
18 Lang, T. *et al*. (1984). op. cit.
19 Lang, T. *et al*. (1984). op. cit.
20 Milburn, J. *et al*. (1987). op. cit.
21 Graham, H. (1987a). 'Women's poverty and caring', in Glendinning, C. and Millar, J. (eds) *Women and Poverty in Britain*. Brighton, Wheatsheaf.
22 Lang, T. *et al*. (1984). op. cit.
23 Graham, H. (1987a). op. cit.
24 Lang, T. *et al*. (1984). op. cit.
25 Burghes, L. (1980). 'Living from hand to mouth: a study of 65 families living on supplementary benefit', *Poverty Pamphlet No. 50*. London, Family Services Unit and Child Poverty Action Group.
26 Mooney, K. (1988). 'A healthy diet – who can afford it?' *The Food Magazine*, vol. 1, 3, autumn.
27 John, B. (1986). *Food and Health – First Report of a Shopping Survey*. Social Health Association.
28 London Food Commission (1985). Cited by Cole-Hamilton, I., Lang, T. (1986). *Tightening Belts: A Report on the Impact of Poverty on Food*. London Food Commission.
29 Graham, H. (1984). *Women, Health and the Family*. Brighton, Wheatsheaf.
30 Whichelow, M. (1987). 'Dietary habits', in Cox, B. D. *et al*. (eds) *The Health and Livestyles Survey*. London, Health Promotion Research Trust.
31 Wilson, G. (1989). 'Family food systems, preventive health and dietary change: a policy to increase the health divide?' *Journal of Social Policy*, vol. 18, April: 2.
32 Charles, N. and Kerr, M. (1987). 'Just the way it is: gender and age differences in

family food consumption', in Brannan, J. and Wilson, G. (eds) *Give and Take in Families: Studies in Resource Distribution*. London, Allen & Unwin.

33 Whichelow, M. (1987). op. cit.
34 Charles, N. and Kerr, M. (1987). op. cit.
35 Wilson, G. (1989). op. cit.
36 Burghes, L. (1980). op. cit.
37 Charles, N. and Kerr, M. (1985). *Attitudes Towards the Feeding and Nutrition of Young Children*, Research Report No. 4, June 1985. London, Health Education Council.
38 Murcott, A. (1982). 'Cooking and the costed: a note on the domestic preparation of meals', in Murcott, A. (ed.) *The Sociology of Food and Eating*. Aldershot, Gower.
39 Charles, N. and Kerr, M. (1985). op. cit.
40 Charles, N. and Kerr, M. (1987). op. cit.
41 Charles, N. and Kerr, M. (1985). op. cit.
42 Whichelow, M. (1987). op. cit.
43 Pahl, J. (1988). 'Earning, sharing, spending: married couples and their money', in Walker, R. and Parker, G. (eds) *Money Matters*. London, Sage.
44 Charles, N. and Kerr, M. (1985). op. cit.
45 Graham, H. (1987b). 'Being poor; perceptions and coping strategies of lone mothers', in Brannen, J. and Wilson, G. (eds) *Give and Take in Families*. London, Allen & Unwin.
46 Charles, N. and Kerr, M. (1985). op cit.
47 Charles, N. and Kerr, M. (1985). op. cit.
48 Charles, N. and Kerr, M. (1985). op. cit.
49 Pahl, J. (1983). 'The allocation of money and the structuring of inequality within marriage' *Sociological Review*, vol. 31: 237-61.
50 Wilson, G. (1987). 'Money: patterns of responsibility and irresponsibility in marriage', in Brannen, J. and Wilson, G. (eds) *Give and Take in Families; Studies in Resource Distribution*. London, Allen & Unwin.
51 Walsh, A. and Lister, R. (1985). *Mothers' Life-Line: A Survey of How Women Use and Value Child Benefits*. London, Child Poverty Action Group.
52 Burghes, L. (1980). op. cit.
53 Graham, H. (1987a). op. cit.
54 Graham, H. (1987a). op. cit.
55 Graham, H. (1987b). op. cit.
56 Graham, H. (1987a). op. cit.
57 Nelson, M. and Naismith, D. (1979). Cited by Cole-Hamilton, I. and Lang, T. (1986). *Tightening Belts: A Report on the Impact of Poverty on Food*. London Food Commission.
58 Garman, A., Chinn, S. and Rona, R. (1982). Cited by Cole-Hamilton, I. (1988). op. cit.
59 Todd, J. E. and Dodd, T. (1985). *Children's Dental Health in the UK*. Office of Population, Censuses and Surveys, London, HMSO.
60 Hackett, A., Rugg-Gunn, A., Appleton, D. *et al.* (1984). 'A two-year longitudinal nutritional survey of 405 Northumberland children initially aged 11.5 years' *British Journal of Nutrition*, 51: 67-75.
61 Wenlock, R. and Dusselduff, M. (1986). *The Diets of British School-children*. London, Department of Health and Social Security.

62 Bull, N. L. (1985). 'Dietary habits of 15–25 year olds' *Human Nutrition, Applied Nutrition*, 39a, Supplement 1, 1–68.

63 Hanes, F. (1986). 'Food and the Fowler reviews'. Cited by Cole-Hamilton, I. (1988). op. cit.

64 Crawford, M., Doyle, W., Craft, I. *et al.* (1986). 'A comparison of food intake during pregnancy and birthweight in high and low socio-economic groups' *Progress in Lipid Research*, vol. 25, Pergamon Press.

65 Pearson, D., Burns, S. and Cunningham, K. (1977). 'Dietary surveys of immigrant school girls in Leicester' *Journal of Human Nutrition*, 31: 362.

66 The Disability Alliance (1988). *Disability Rights Handbook*, 13th edition, April 1988–April 1989, Disability Alliance Education and Research Association.

67 London Borough of Camden (1985). 'Board and lodging; effect of new regulations on non-priority claimants, report of the Director of Housing'. Cited by Cole-Hamilton, I. (1988). op. cit.

68 Health Visitor Association/Shelter Survey, cited by Drennan, V. and Stearn, J., 'Health visitors and homeless families' *Health Visitor Journal*, November, vol. 59: 340–2.

69 Conway, J. (ed.) (1988). *Prescription for Poor Health: The Crisis for Homeless Families*. London, London Food Commission; Maternity Alliance; Shac; Shelter.

70 Wilson, G. (1989). op. cit.

4 | HOUSING CONDITIONS AND HEALTH

INTRODUCTION

The quality of our home environment has an important bearing on our quality of life. Most people spend at least half of their waking hours at home. Some groups such as mothers and young children, carers, unemployed, sick and disabled people spend substantially longer periods at home each day. Our home environment not only has an important effect on our quality of life, it also has a pervasive effect on our health and our relationships with other people. Housing is, therefore, a major health resource. Housing can protect individuals from physical and mental ill health. Alternatively it can increase their vulnerability, depending on the standard, location, and type of accommodation they live in. Like food and eating, poor housing affects health directly through physiological processes, and indirectly through behavioural and psychological processes. Housing conditions also help or hinder parents, particularly mothers, in their role as carers. For parents living on the breadline, parenting in poor housing becomes an even more arduous task. Homes can be a major source of personal wealth. They can be used for investment or collateral or as a way of passing on wealth. In this sense, housing is a key resource that can mediate a family's access to other health resources, such as leisure, transport and health-care facilities. Furthermore, housing is also a marker of social status and a marker of social mobility.

Access to healthy homes, like many other health resources, depends on income, social class, age group, geographical region, ethnic group and gender. Comfortable and pleasant housing conditions are not universally enjoyed in Britain, nor equally distributed among the population. Poverty and housing are inextricably linked, with the poorest and most vulnerable members of the population living in the least desirable housing conditions. Studies suggest that housing inequalities undoubtedly contribute to the relative inequalities in health that have been clearly documented.[1,2]

In the last decade many politicians and policy-makers have disputed claims that have linked health with housing conditions, preferring to blame aspects of individual behaviour instead. The greater frequency of respiratory symptoms among occupants of damp housing has been blamed on smoking behaviour, or the irresponsible behaviour of occupants who fail to allow adequate ventilation or heating, and who should refrain from drying washing indoors. This situation has not been helped by researchers who have found it difficult to establish the nature of the relationship between housing and health. This is because people who live in unhealthy homes usually suffer other forms of social and economic disadvantage, making it difficult to disentangle the effects of housing conditions from other factors.[3] However, a number of recent research studies have shed some light on how aspects of the home environment have a direct effect on physical and mental health, causing a multiple of health problems. This chapter will explore the relationship between poverty, poor housing conditions, and health by examining:

- *Housing patterns:* examining tenure patterns and type and standard of accommodation according to income, family structure, gender and ethnic group.
- *Housing and fuel costs.*
- *The relationship between housing conditions and family health:* highlighting the problems of damp, overcrowding, poor layout and design and inhospitable geographical locations for family health.

HOUSING PATTERNS: WHERE DO LOW-INCOME FAMILIES LIVE?

There can be little doubt that housing conditions have improved dramatically, in an absolute sense, in the twentieth century. For example, in 1986, 98 per cent of all houses in Britain had the unshared use of a bath or shower and had an inside toilet.[4] Data from the censuses and OPCS paint an optimistic picture of housing conditions in Britain in the 1980s. Yet these data do not accurately reflect the extent of contemporary poor housing conditions. They do not, for example, reflect the extent of structural and disrepair problems. Nor do they reflect the fact that certain groups in society experience poor housing conditions relative to others. Furthermore, it has been suggested that returns from local authorities, who provide the bulk of data on housing conditions, underestimate the extent of housing problems that exists in Britain today.[5]

TABLE 4.1 Tenure by ethnic group

Household	Tenure type			
	Owner occupied %	Council rented %	Private rented %	Housing association %
White	59	30	9	2
West Indian	41	46	6	8
Indian	77	16	5	2
Pakistani	80	13	5	1
Bangladeshi	30	53	11	4
African/Asian	73	19	5	2

Source: Brown, C. (1984). *Black and White Britain*, Third Study Policy Studies Institute

TENURE PATTERNS

Housing tenure is a valuable indicator of housing quality. It acts as a surrogate indicator for a number of other factors such as building standards, housing type, security and location. For example, building standards are generally higher in the owner-occupied sector than in the rented sector. Tenure is also related to type of accommodation. Owner occupiers are much more likely to live in detached or semi-detached houses than flats or terraced houses. In this case, tenure also gives some indication of the amount of living space a family might have. Families living in flats are far less likely to have as much living space as families living in detached houses. Owner-occupied accommodation is also likely to be in more desirable residential areas, and to be more secure than rented housing. Later in this chapter, we will see that these are important factors relating to the health of occupants.

If patterns of tenure are examined, it is possible to see striking differences between social groups.

Housing tenure is strongly related to household income. Data from the General Household Survey, 1986[6] indicates that the majority of households in the lowest income group live in rented accommodation, mainly in the local authority/new town sector. Only 34 per cent of low-income households are owner occupiers. Among households with the highest income, the majority (87 per cent) are owner occupiers.

Housing tenure is closely related to household composition and gender. Two-parent families are far more likely to live in owner-occupied housing than lone-parent families (see figure 4.1), reflecting their greater economic prosperity. As we saw in chapter 1, lone-parent families are likely to have lower household incomes than two-parent families. As a result, lone parents depend heavily on the public sector for their housing. This is particularly the case for families headed by lone mothers. Burnell and Wadworth's study[7] of children in lone-parent families found that, while 42

FIGURE 4.1   Housing tenure and one- and two-parent families, 1986

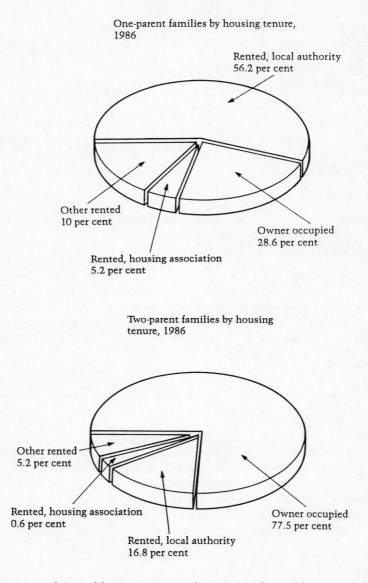

One-parent families by housing tenure, 1986

Rented, local authority
56.2 per cent

Other rented
10 per cent

Rented, housing association
5.2 per cent

Owner occupied
28.6 per cent

Two-parent families by housing tenure, 1986

Other rented
5.2 per cent

Rented, housing association
0.6 per cent

Rented, local authority
16.8 per cent

Owner occupied
77.5 per cent

Source: National Council for One-Parent Families (1989). *70th Annual Report*. London, National Council for One-Parent Families.

per cent of lone-father households lived in owner-occupied accommodation, only 23 per cent of lone-mother families lived in this type of accommodation. Housing tenure is often affected by divorce. This occurs predominantly in the owner-occupied sector, when one or both partners are forced to move into rented housing due to the sale of the family home in a divorce settlement, or the inability of the remaining parent to afford the cost of the home. One in two of all divorced or separated women have their housing needs met by the local authority.[8]

Housing tenure is also related to 'race' and ethnic group. The most valuable information on 'race' and housing comes from Brown's survey of the social and economic circumstances of West Indian and Asian families in Britain (see table 4.1). As table 4.1 suggests, tenure profiles differ significantly between minority ethnic groups, particularly between Asian and Afro-Caribbean groups. This is related to the different immigration patterns, immigration policies and labour-market opportunities experienced by individual minority ethnic groups (for an in-depth analysis see Luthera 1989).[9] Owner occupancy is most common among Pakistani, Indian, African-Asian and white households; with West Indian and Bangladeshi households least likely to be owner occupiers. Unfortunately we have no information on the tenure patterns of other ethnic groups, such as Chinese and Irish households. West Indian and Bangladeshi households are most likely to be council tenants. Housing associations are an important source of housing for Afro-Caribbean households, with 8 per cent, compared to 2 per cent of white households, living in housing-association properties.

The general trend in housing tenure is towards increasing home ownership.[10] The number of owner-occupied homes has doubled between 1961 and 1987 in the UK, to 14.5 million. This represents 66 per cent of the total housing stock.[11] While a growing number of households are choosing to buy their homes, many low-income families do not have this choice. As we shall see later in this chapter, housing costs are generally higher for owner occupiers and beyond the budget of low-income families.

The amount of private property available for rent has declined over the last two decades, increasing the demand for council housing. Changing marriage and divorce patterns and an increase in the number of households who have been evicted due to mortgage default and rent arrears have further increased the demand for council housing in the last decade. However, this increased demand has been accompanied by a decline in the number of council properties available for rent. The net result is a shortage of homes.

The decline in the amount of council homes available for rent is associated with the Housing Act (1985). This Act, based on the Conservative Government's policy to promote home ownership and reduce the role of the state in housing, gives council tenants the right to buy their homes from the local authority. It has been calculated that between 1980 and 1987, one million council homes were sold under 'right to buy' legislation.[12] Changes to housing finance legislation have made it increasingly difficult for local authorities to use the proceeds of council house sales to build more homes for rent. Housing policy was further modified by the Housing Act, 1988, which abolished the 'fair rent' scheme for all new tenancies after January 1989, allowing private landlords to charge market rates. Critics have argued that market rents are unlikely to increase the number of properties available for rent in the private sector. This Act also allows council tenants to choose a landlord other than the local authority. It remains to be seen whether choosing an alternative landlord will improve the housing conditions of tenants. Furthermore, changes to housing association finance provision under the Housing Act, 1988, reduce government subsidies to housing associations, forcing them to use private-sector finance. It has been suggested that this will increase housing-association rents substantially, thus limiting the ability of housing associations to help low-income households who have traditionally formed the tenant group of housing associations.

The decline in the amount of private property for rent has hit families who live in rural areas particularly hard. In many rural areas council properties for rent are scarce and house prices high, forcing those who cannot afford to buy their homes to move to urban areas or resort to tied accommodation, 'winter lets' or caravan accommodation – the 'true ghettos of the rural poor'.[13] For many low-income families in rural areas, being a tenant goes hand in hand with insecure tenancy and decaying and sub-standard property.

A decline in the availability of public and private rented housing and changes in social-security legislation affecting young people have substantially increased the number of homeless people in the UK. Under the Housing (Homeless Persons) Act, 1985, local authorities have a statutory duty to provide accommodation for homeless families in 'priority need': households with pregnant women, dependent children or people who are vulnerable through age or disability.

 In 1987, local authorities in England and Wales accepted responsibility to rehouse 118,000 households, of which 107,000 were classed as 'in priority need'[14] compared to a total of 96,000 households 'in priority need' in 1981, when local authorities accepted responsibility to rehouse 74,000 households.

However, these figures do not reflect the true extent of the homelessness problem. Under the Housing (Homeless Persons) Act, 1985, local authorities are not obliged to accept the responsibility to rehouse households who become 'intentionally' homeless or individuals who do not fall into the 'priority need' category: single people or childless couples. These groups are required to find their own accommodation. An increase in the number of single people sleeping on the streets, as inhabitants of 'cardboard cities', is a testimony to the problem of housing shortages.

Those families most at risk of homelessness are those who suffer other social and economic disadvantage: low-income families, large families, lone-parent households and Black and minority ethnic groups. In addition, a growing number of young, single people are increasingly found among the homeless.

 In 1987 78 per cent of homeless households in priority need contained a pregnant woman or dependent children.[15]

In 1986 Black households made up 40 per cent of those families accepted as homeless in London.[16]

A reduction in the availability of local-authority housing stock means that a growing number of homeless families are having to spend a period of time in temporary accommodation: hotels, hostels and short-term lets. From 1981–7, the number of households living in temporary accommodation more than doubled.[17] And as the availability of local-authority accommodation has declined, the length of time that families have had to spend in temporary accommodation has become progressively longer.[18] This has an important knock-on effect on access to local-authority housing for families who already have homes but who are waiting to be rehoused because of substandard amenities, overcrowding, racist attacks or medical reasons.

TYPE AND STANDARD OF ACCOMMODATION

Differences in housing patterns are not restricted to differences in tenure. Good standard accommodation is not universally available or shared out equally between social groups.

Low-income families are housed in poorer quality accommodation than their better-off counterparts. While there is a lack of recent data on income and housing standards, it is clear that higher-income families can afford to pay for larger and better-quality housing. They can pay to keep their property in a good structural condition. However, low income means that poor families have very little choice about the type or standard of accommodation they occupy.

Low-income families are more likely to live in flats and terraced houses than higher-income groups. These properties tend to have the least living space and the worst structural and disrepair problems (see figure 4.2).

Whilst the structural condition of Britain's housing stock today is, without doubt, better than that of the early twentieth century, recent studies of housing conditions have indicated that housing policies have failed to provide continued improvements in the structure of Britain's housing stock.[19] Although the number of properties lacking basic amenities, such as unshared use of a bath or toilet, has decreased, the number of properties in a state of disrepair has not declined and, according to some researchers,[20] is actually growing.

FIGURE 4.2 Type of dwelling by usual weekly gross income of head of household

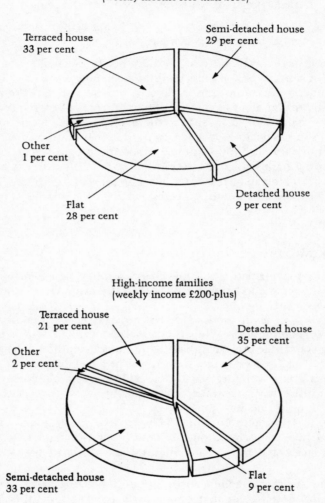

Low-income families
(weekly income less than £100)

Terraced house
33 per cent

Semi-detached house
29 per cent

Other
1 per cent

Flat
28 per cent

Detached house
9 per cent

High-income families
(weekly income £200-plus)

Terraced house
21 per cent

Detached house
35 per cent

Other
2 per cent

Semi-detached house
33 per cent

Flat
9 per cent

Source: Office of Population Census and Surveys (1989). *General Household Survey*, 1987. London, HMSO.

25 per cent of Britain's housing stock is either unfit for habitation, lacking amenities or in a state of disrepair.[21]

Data from the English House Condition Survey, 1986, indicates that low-income groups frequently live in housing that has the worst disrepair problems and structural faults:

Half of all households lacking amenities and one-third of all those in unfit housing had very low net incomes of less than £3000 per year.[22]

Low-income families who own or are buying their own homes are frequently concentrated in pre-1919 housing, in inner cities and industrial towns. These properties often have substantial structural problems or are in a state of disrepair, for example, needing a new roof or beset by damp problems. Low availability of repair grants and low incomes mean that repairs are beyond the budget of many families. In recent years this situation has been aggravated by the fact that house prices have risen rapidly, often faster than earnings. This means that many parents, particularly in the South-east, are faced with very high mortgage repayments at a time when the presence of children is stretching resources to the limit.

Desrepair and structural faults are also problems for families living in public-sector rented accommodation, an important source of housing for low-income groups. While the private sector continued to use tried and tested construction methods and designs, local-authority building pro- grammes pioneered the use of new materials and modern designs. The result is that many properties built in the 1950s and 1960s have frequently proved to be unsuitable housing for the very people they were meant to house. Many of these properties, particularly the large number of high-rise flats that were built, have design and construction faults. The problems associated with high-rise flats epitomize many of the problems associated with public-sector housing: damp and condensation problems, poor heat and sound insulation and lack of private access and safe play space for children. Many of these blocks are now viewed as unsuitable for families with young children. The effect of these housing conditions on health will be discussed later in this chapter. A significant number of these properties now need demolishing or repairing. Yet changes to local–authority finance provision means that local authorities are finding it increasingly difficult to finance repair and maintenance costs or replace unsuitable housing stock. In 1984 local authorities estimated that 84 per cent of their stock needed some kind of renovation. The average cost of repairs per property amounted to £4,900.[23]

A disproportionate number of Black families live in substandard accom- modation. Data on the housing situation of Black families indicates that Black families are more likely than white families to live in poor housing:

Brown's study (1984) of the living circumstances of Black families found that they are twice as likely as white families to be in flats, and have higher levels of overcrowding.[24]

The English House Condition Survey, 1986, estimated that households whose heads identified themselves as being born in the New Commonwealth or Pakistan are 2.5 times more likely to be living in unfit housing than other households.[25]

Black families who wish to buy their own homes are often forced to purchase older properties in poor, declining areas. Not only are repair and renovation costs likely to be beyond the reach of low-income Black families, but the quality and the value of the equity held by Black families is disproportionately low and prone to devaluation.[26] Many Black families live in the least saleable portions of the housing stock (run-down terraced housing and council properties), and thus have little opportunity to increase capital assets through house sales.

Several studies have highlighted how racial discrimination affects local housing allocation and exchange systems. Studies for the Commission for Racial Equality indicate that Black families living in public-sector rented accommodation tend to be allocated smaller properties and flats (particularly flats on the upper floors of high-rise blocks) more frequently than white families, irrespective of household composition.[27,28] Black families are also more likely than white families to be housed in high-density areas of Britain's inner cities, and in areas where labour markets and local economies are less secure.[29]

Women and children bear the brunt of poor housing standards. In all tenures, women and children are likely to experience the worst housing.[30] First, women and children usually spend longer periods at home than men, and thus are more likely to be exposed to the hazards of poor housing. Second, women's economic disadvantage means that female-headed households, which frequently contain children, have difficulty paying for decent housing and are more likely than men to be housed in the sectors that have the worst construction and disrepair problems: private and public rented housing. Thus the decline in the number of private and public sector properties for rent and rising rents in both sectors have had the most severe impact on women and their children.

The Glasgow House Condition Survey indicated that children and teenagers are likely to be in poorer housing than any other group.[31]

The London Research Centre's survey found that two-thirds of the homeless are women.[32]

Women with violent partners have found themselves hard hit by recent housing policies. A shortfall in council properties has meant that women may have no option but to stay with a violent partner, as the chance of

FIGURE 4.3   Housing and fuel costs as a proportion of weekly household expenditure, 1987

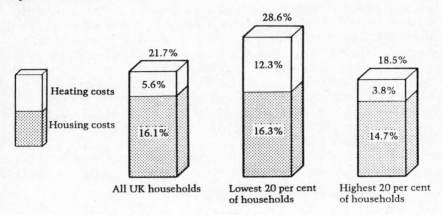

Source: Department of employment (1989). *Employment Gazette*, May 1989.

alternative accommodation being available is low. Women who have been able to find a place in a refuge find it virtually impossible to be rehoused into council properties. This has created bottlenecks in many refuges. Furthermore, changes to housing-benefit legislation have made it difficult for women to claim the full cost of hostel or refuge accommodation from local authorities.

HOUSING PATTERNS: WHAT DO LOW-INCOME FAMILIES PAY?

Weekly housing costs are usually highest for households who are buying their homes with a mortgage, although these households are accumulating a capital asset at the same time.[33] As a consequence, home ownership is frequently beyond the budget of low-income families. However, irrespective of type of tenure, housing costs, like food costs, account for a larger proportion of the total weekly expenditure of low-income families than of higher-income families (see figure 4.3).

Rented accommodation is no longer the cheap housing option that it used to be. Deregulation of rents in the private sector and rises in council-house rents mean that the cost of housing has risen for many low-income families. This has been compounded by changes to housing-benefit legislation. The housing-benefit scheme has become less generous since the early 1980s, as the maximum qualifying income for housing benefit has been reduced. Moreover, the Housing Act, 1988, gives rent officers the power to impose a rent ceiling for benefit purposes. Local authorities can pay over the ceiling if they wish to, but they then lose any central government subsidy. Thus families who rely on housing benefit, because of low income, may have to find an extra amount from the household budget. Furthermore, the introduction of the community charge, or poll tax as it is more commonly known, has increased the living costs of low-income families. Although this is a tax on people and not on property like the rates system it replaces, poll-tax bills indicate that many households in the low- and middle-income range will have to pay more under the new system than the old, despite the existence of a rebate system. Although the poll tax will be replaced by a new charge in the mid-1990s, it remains to be seen whether low-income families will be any better off under a new system.

Since 1979 there has been a rise in the number of households with housing-related debts. On the basis of a study on credit and debt in the UK, Berthoud et al. (1990)[34] estimated that:

> 1 million tenants (16 per cent of all tenants) are in arrears with their rent

> 250,000 mortgage holders (3 per cent of all mortgage holders) are behind with mortgage payments.

This confirms other research findings that suggest that family costs rise with family size. Berthoud et al. found that debt problems appear to increase with family size and to be linked to changes in household structure: births, deaths and marriage or relationship breakdown. There is no evidence to suggest that the increase in debt is related to the increase in the amount of consumer credit.[35]

Fuel costs are closely related to the housing conditions of low-income families. If low income affects housing 'choice', it also affects the 'choice' of fuel for many families. While a family which is buying a home may choose to avoid purchasing a property with an expensive source of heating, such as electric central heating, a council tenant is forced to accept what she/he is offered, regardless of the effectiveness or efficiency of the fuel source. The fact that many low-income families are confined to housing that is badly designed and built, and/or in a poor state of repair means that fuel bills may be increased through damp and condensation problems and poor insulation. Together with housing costs, fuel costs account for a significant part of the weekly household expenditure for low-income families (see figure 4.3). Fuel costs account for a greater proportion of the expenditure of low-income families than higher-income families.

Studies of how low-income families budget indicate that housing and fuel costs are frequently paid first, before food or other family expenses.[36] There has been a growing tendency for the housing and fuel costs of families on social-security benefit to be recovered directly from benefit, before they reach the claimant. Although this ensures that bills are paid, it leaves the budget-holder with less control over weekly income and expenditure and less opportunity to budget for other household expenses.

Fuel costs are a major source of debt for low-income families. In 1987, 90,000 electricity users and 60,000 gas users were disconnected due to debt.[37] While the rate of electricity disconnections has remained steady since 1981, the rate of gas disconnections has increased rapidly. Lone parents and families with children are over-represented among those with fuel-debt problems and are therefore likely to form a significant proportion of households without fuel for a period each year. As women and children spend longer periods in the home than men, they suffer disproportionately from both fuel economy and fuel disconnections. Although electricity and gas boards say they are sensitive to households with children, disconnections still occur. Households may also be disconnected where household appliances are deemed to be unsafe, leaving families who cannot afford to replace equipment without any means of cooking or heating.

HOUSING CONDITIONS AND PATTERNS OF HEALTH

We have seen how low-income families are more likely to live in housing that is badly designed, poorly constructed and in a state of disrepair. The consequence is that many low-income families have to live in damp, noisy, overcrowded accommodation that is associated with physical and mental health problems and increased accident rates in adults and children. While some housing problems affect the health of any occupant, others are only likely to be harmful to individuals or families with certain physical, social or health characteristics.

There is a close statistical correlation between housing tenure and health. The research indicates that owner occupiers are likely to have the lowest death rates and council tenants the highest death rates. Studies have shown how certain aspects of physical and mental ill health are associated with tenure. For example:

> Kogevinas's study (1990) of social factors and cancer survival rates suggests an association between deaths from cancer and housing tenure. This study showed that male council-house tenants were more likely to die from cancer of the face, oesophagus, stomach, larynx, bladder and lung, and women tenants were especially more likely to die from cancer of the cervix, than owner occupiers.[38]

The close association between tenure and death rates is explicable in terms of the fact that tenure, as well as being a proxy indicator of income and class, is an indicator of the type and standard of housing a family will experience. In this sense the association between housing tenure and death rates is likely to reflect the fact that families who live in rented accommodation experience not only the adverse effects of low income and poor working conditions but also more damp, overcrowding, noise and design problems and live in less desirable locations than owner occupiers. It is to these aspects that this chapter now turns.

Damp is a major health hazard and the result of poor structural maintenance, design and construction. The problems are further exacerbated for low-income families who may not be able to afford the costs of heating their homes adequately. It is a major housing problem faced by many families, particularly those living in public-sector rented accommodation or older properties. A number of studies have attempted to establish a relationship between damp and ill health. Some of these studies have been criticized as lacking scientific rigour or displaying methodological flaws. The contention is that such studies have been unable to show that the greater frequency of respiratory symptoms among families in damp housing is related to the damp itself rather than aspects of individual behaviour, such as smoking. There have also been attempts by policy-makers to redefine damp problems as condensation problems, related to the behaviour of residents, rather than a consequence of structural defects. For example, failure to allow adequate ventilation, failure to heat properties properly or drying clothes indoors have all been used as explanations. However, the findings from Platt *et al.*'s study, which overcame many of the methodological flaws of previous studies, indicated that there is a direct relationship between damp and mould growth and the health of residents:[39]

 Adults living in damp and mouldy housing were likely to report more symptoms, such as nausea, blocked nose, breathlessness, backache and fainting, than people living in dry housing conditions.

 Children living in damp and mouldy housing had a greater number of respiratory symptoms, such as wheeziness, runny nose and sore throats, as well as headaches and fever, and irritability than children living in dry housing.

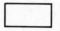 The number of symptoms increased with increasing exposure to severe damp and mould growth.

 These differences between people living in damp or dry conditions persisted when smoking behaviour, income, unemployment and overcrowding were controlled for.

This study also highlights how physical ill health can affect psychological well-being and behaviour. Both children and adults who were exposed to high levels of damp and mould growth had higher levels of irritability and 'bad nerves' than their counterparts in similar, but dry housing. Physical symptoms can cause irritability, depression, and unhappiness, which are reflected in an individual's behaviour, for example, temper outbursts in a child or a low level of patience in a parent of a young child. For children it is likely that damp-related ill health may be compounded by the fact that ill children are unable to attend school or nursery as frequently as other children. This in turn may hinder a child's developmental progress.

Overcrowding was recognized as a health hazard as early as the nineteenth century and is probably the most well-researched housing factor. Research indicates that overcrowding is associated with a number of physical and mental health problems in adults and children: respiratory and digestive-tract infections, depression, stress and psychological distress.[40,41,42] Living in overcrowded housing makes it difficult for individuals to control the amount of social contact they have with other members of the family. Lack of privacy, lack of space to store personal belongings and constant contact with other people are likely to increase stress and domestic tensions. Tension may be difficult to diffuse where individuals are unable to find personal space or move to a quiet room to calm down. Lack of space and the tension it creates are likely to affect the quality of both parental relationships and parent–child relationships. Living in an overcrowded home may make it very difficult for parents to carry out their parenting role and meet their children's needs. Creating the domestic conditions necessary for maintaining good health, such as quiet sleeping arrangements, and hygienic cooking and food preparation facilities, is difficult, if not impossible, where space is limited. Moreover, it may be physically and/or emotionally hard, or even impossible, to carry out advice from health and welfare workers. For example, a parent in a crowded home may find it impossible to introduce the night-time routine that the family health visitor advises because the child shares a bedroom with other children.

Poor layout and design of homes has also been shown to be associated with health problems. The design and layout of flats and maisonettes have attracted the most attention, particularly the experience of living above ground level. Flats have frequently been used to house families with young children, particularly in the public sector, although many local authorities now have a policy of not allocating properties on upper floors of high-rise blocks to families with young children. Flat-living has been associated with a number of health problems:

> Children who live in flats have higher incidences of respiratory infections than children who live in houses.[43]

> People who live in flats have higher incidences of emotional disturbances and mental-health problems.[44]

Some of these problems are likely to be associated with the fact that, on average, flats are 50 per cent smaller than houses[45] and are often more crowded. They also tend to have worse design and structural faults. Flat dwellers are often exposed to damp and crowding problems. The design of high-rise flats is a source of stress, particularly for parents who live with the fear that their children will fall from a window or balcony of a high-rise block, fall on the stairs, or injure themselves in the lifts or on the fire escape. Several studies have shown how parental concern about child safety among flat residents causes high levels of anxiety.[46,47] This may partly explain why women who live in flats experience high levels of nervous disorders. Studies of flat-residents also draw attention to the fact that design features such as interconnecting walkways and lack of control over space outside the front door can be damaging to a resident's sense of well-being. Coleman's large-scale study[48] of social malaise among residents of flats and houses found that the degree of social malaise (indicated by the level of care of communal areas, graffiti and vandalism) increased in blocks of flats where residents had no control over the entrance to their dwelling. The potential for racial attacks is also increased in these types of dwellings. While housing type and design clearly have an important bearing on the health of families, other studies have highlighted how the location of a dwelling can affect residents' level of satisfaction with their housing circumstances and the number of illness symptoms they report.

Poor design and layout are also problems that are frequently faced by people with disabilities and their families. Many homes are unsuitable for people with physical disabilities. Rooms may be too small for wheelchairs to manoeuvre or carers to assist a person with daily living activities. Access into and out of the house and to upstairs rooms may be difficult for people with disabilities, unless homes have adequate adaptations. For families with people with mental or learning disabilities, homes that do not have secure gardens, or window fastenings, to prevent a person's wandering off may be a problem. Moreover, people with severe disabilities are likely to need a room of their own, both for their peace, and to allow other family members some respite from caring. Glendinning's survey found that housing layout, design and space problems are common among families with children with disabilities, with half of the respondents reporting housing difficulties.[49]

Cramped living conditions and poorly designed housing are both related to high home accident rates among children. The Child Accident Prevention Trust estimates that 250,000 childhood accidents a year are due to bad housing design.[50] Home accidents are the commonest cause of death to children over one year of age. Crowded living areas, poor lighting on communal stairways, badly designed kitchens, fittings, and balconies expose children to the risk of accidents more frequently than conditions in better housing. Moreover, these conditions make it more physically and mentally difficult for parents to protect their children from hazards within the home. For example, a small, badly designed kitchen makes if difficult for parents to cook safely and supervise children at the same time. For many parents in this situation the options are either to allow the child into the kitchen to play during food preparation and cooking; to leave the child to play unsupervised in another room; or to restrain the child, usually in a pram and against his or her will, within view of the parent. Each of these options has either a safety risk or is so stress-inducing that it may be impossible to carry out. And for many parents, the opportunity to allow a child to play outdoors instead of inside an unsafe home is not available. Low-income families often live in locations where the outdoors offers little protection to children. Areas with busy roads, no confined safe play areas, no gardens, and hazards such as broken glass, discarded rubbish, and dog excreta, are the only play areas for many children who live in inner cities and run-down urban areas.

Geographical location has an important influence on mental and physical health, particularly the health of children. Low-income families, especially one-parent families and Black families are much more likely to be housed in neighbourhoods that are unattractive, densely populated, with poorly maintained houses and communal areas, and poor amenities. Byrne *et al.*'s study[51] of 'difficult to let' council estates illustrates the importance of housing location for health. This study found that residents who lived in these areas reported high rates of dissatisfaction with their housing circumstances and more ill health than residents of other council estates:

47 per cent of children living in 'difficult to let' areas had frequent chesty coughs compared to 27 per cent of children from other council estates.

In every age group, except for over 65s, people who lived in 'difficult to let' areas experienced more psychological distress than people from more desirable council housing areas. This was associated with location and not housing type.

Although health differences existed between house and flat dwellers, these were not statistically significant. However, consistent differences were found between dwellings of the same type and standard, which could be explained in terms of where they were located. 'Difficult to let' housing areas were in less desirable locations, had poorer environments and were not as well maintained. Thus 'bad' housing did not necessarily conform to the stereotype of high-rise blocks or non-traditional design.

Where we live determines our access to other vital health resources. Townsend[52] argues that we need a concept of 'environmental poverty' which would refer to lack of, or lack of access to, gardens, parks, play space, shopping facilities and health centres, as well as taking account of exposure to pollution such as noise and dirt. Many low-income families are housed in inner-city areas and urban housing complexes on the outskirts of large towns and cities, where 'environmental poverty' abounds. Poor access to community provision such as playgroups and nurseries, social and recreational facilities, shops that sell healthy foods, safe play areas and health services, and transport systems that inhibit movement out of the area make childcare a difficult task for parents who are already coping with the burden of living on the breadline. Studies of 'difficult to let' and high-density housing in Liverpool and the Wirral concluded that infections could also be traced to the unhygienic food vans which were used in the vicinity, because of a lack of food shops; poor refuse disposal; and drying clothes indoors due to lack of outdoor facilities.[53,54]

From this information it is clear that housing conditions strongly influence child-rearing practices. However, much health and welfare work with families with young children is based on an approach that identifies child-rearing problems with the behaviour of parents rather than the problems that housing factors pose for them. Thus 'advice' to parents consists largely of suggestions that parents change aspects of their behaviour rather than focusing information or action to assist parents to relieve, challenge or change the effect of poor housing circumstances. Child accident-prevention work illustrates this point well. Higher home-accident rates among children from poorer social groups are frequently blamed on the failure of parents to supervise and care adequately for their children, failing to take account of the fact that conditions inside and outside home have a strong influence on the behaviour of both the parent and the child.

Homelessness appears to be a health hazard that is on the increase. Surveys of the living conditions of families in hotel accommodation, and of their health status indicate that the conditions they experience threaten their health and safety. Hotel accommodation is often overcrowded, insanitary and lacking the basic amenities for good health:

A survey by the Department of the Environment found that 38 per cent of multi-occupied dwellings lacked satisfactory means of escape from fire, 33 per cent needed major repairs, 28 per cent lacked proper amenities and 16 per cent were overcrowded.[55]

Insanitary conditions and overcrowding result in higher levels of infectious diseases and vomiting and diarrhoeal illnesses. Dampness and overcrowding are probably the cause of high levels of respiratory-tract infections in children in hotel accommodation. Poor access to cooking facilities and the extra food expenses that homelessness bring lead to nutritional problems (see chapter 3). High accident rates among children living in hotel accommodation have been noted in a number of studies.[56,57] Hotel and hostel conditions make it difficult for parents to keep children safe. Cramped rooms, non-secure windows, steep staircases and unguarded electrical appliances (particularly kettles on the floor) place children at high risk of physical injury. In addition to the risk of injury from accidents, parents with children in hotel accommodation have also expressed their fear that other residents and visitors to the hotel may place their children's safety at risk. Studies have also indicated that children living in temporary accommodation suffer emotionally and educationally, as well as physically.

Behaviour problems such as over-activity, temper tantrums, bed wetting and soiling and aggressive behaviour are common. Lack of space to play and do homework can result in speech, gross motor and learning delays. The stress of living in temporary accommodation also appears to affect the mental health of parents. Anxiety, depression and problems in maintaining personal relationships have all been shown to be common in homeless adults. Living in temporary accommodation frequently involves a move out of the family's neighbourhood, rupturing social and family support networks, and resulting in changes in schools and playgroups. At a time when many families need additional social and emotional support, it is often least available.

> Research in Bayswater found that 40 per cent of children living in hotel accommodation had behavioural problems.[58]

> Conway's study of families in hotel accommodation found high levels of stress and depression among mothers.[59]

The high incidence of ill health among homeless parents and children is often exacerbated by poor access to primary health care. Families in temporary accommodation often fail to register with a general practitioner in the vicinity of their temporary home, in the belief that they will be moved to a permanent home in the near future. Those who do seek to register with a general practitioner may only be able to do so as temporary residents, in which case their medical records remain with their previous family doctor. Thus immunization and screening check records are often not available, and immunization and screening programmes are rarely completed. Failure to receive adequate information from housing officers about the location of families makes it difficult for health visitors and midwives to trace homeless families to offer health care. Moreover, health and welfare workers are failing to offer services that are required due to heavy workloads.

CONCLUSION AND IMPLICATIONS FOR PRACTICE

The data on housing patterns in the UK indicate that housing inequality remains today. It is clear that absolute and relative housing inequality exists. Some households experience housing conditions that fall below an absolute standard, according to an officially recognized minimum standard. Other households may not live in housing conditions that fall below a minimum standard but may experience housing conditions that are poor relative to the rest of society. Absolute and relative housing inequality are experienced disproportionately by the poorest and most vulnerable members of society: lone-parent families, families on low income, Black and minority ethnic families, women, people with disabilities, older adults and young single people (although the experiences of the latter two groups are beyond the brief of this book). A growing number of families have no home of their own and there is every indication that the number of homeless families will remain high for some considerable time.

Housing and health are inextricably linked. Studies on the relationship between housing and health indicate that health inequalities are closely linked to housing inequalities. But while some studies have been able to indicate a direct relationship between certain housing conditions and health, other studies have only been able to indicate a close link rather than a causal relationship. Nevertheless, the evidence is strong enough to argue that the housing situation of many households should be improved on health grounds. In addition, housing inequalities are a vehicle for the transmission of other inequalities, such as those in education and leisure and, in particular, inequalities in the ability to accumulate wealth and gain access to credit. For these reasons, it is important to argue for a reduction in housing inequalities on social as well as health grounds.

While housing conditions have a direct physiological effect on health, they clearly affect health through psychological and behavioural processes. As we have seen, poor housing conditions affect the ability of families to care adequately for their health. Yet health and welfare workers continue to work with families from the assumption that people's health behaviour is unrelated to the social and economic context of people's lives. Approaches that focus on changing the behaviour of individuals are unlikely to reduce health problems that stem from poor housing conditions. For many health and welfare workers this fact may foster feelings of helplessness rather than a desire to change to more pro-active approaches. But all fieldworkers have the scope to monitor the housing conditions of clients, to pass this information up and across organizations, as a way of putting the issue back on the agenda. Health and welfare workers can also support local people to gain access to local planning mechanisms. Local housing schemes need to take on board what local people say they want and need in terms of housing and local facilities, rather than excluding them from decisions.

Health and welfare workers have the opportunity to work toward the provision of community resources that help to mitigate or reduce the effect of poor housing on health. The health of many children and parents may benefit through the provision of more playgroups, nurseries, safe play areas, and through the opportunity to meet and receive support from others with similar housing problems (for example, through women's support groups). The health needs of families who live in poor housing, particularly homeless families, warrant special consideration. Local health services need to look at how they can reduce the barriers that prevent those with the most health needs from using them. Families need access to health services that are responsive to their particular needs, easy to use and welcoming. Finally, fieldworkers need to demonstrate to parents that they understand the context within which parents care for their own and their children's health and well-being, to show they understand the constraints under which families live and care.

REFERENCES

1 Townsend, P. and Davidson, N. (1982). *Inequalities in Health (The Black Report)*. Harmondsworth, Penguin.
2 Whitehead, M. (1987). *The Health Divide: Inequalities in Health in the 1980's*. London, Health Education Council.
3 Smith, A. and Jacobson, B. (1988). *The Nation's Health: A Strategy for the 1990's*. London, King's Fund/Oxford University Press.
4 Office of Populations, Censuses and Surveys (1989). *The General Household Survey, 1986*. London, HMSO.
5 Kemp, P. (1989). 'The housing question', in Herbert, D. and Smith, D. (eds) *Social Problems and the City*. New York, Oxford University Press.
6 Office of Populations, Censuses and Surveys (1989). op. cit.
7 Burnell, I. and Wadsworth, J. (1981). *Children in One-Parent Families*. University of Bristol, Child Health Research Unit.
8 Morris, J. (1988). 'Keeping women in their place' *Roof*, July/August: 20–1.
9 Luthera, M. (1989). 'Race, community, housing and the state – a historical overview', in Bhat, A., *et al.* (eds) *Britain's Black Population*, 2nd edition. Aldershot, Gower.
10 Office of Populations, Censuses and Surveys (1989). *General Household Survey, 1987*. London, HMSO.
11 Central Statistical Office (1989). *Social Trends*. London, HMSO.
12 Central Statistical Office (1989). *ibid.*
13 Lakin, A. (1979). 'Rural housing and housing needs', in Shaw, J. M. (ed.) *Rural Deprivation and Planning*. Norwich, Geo Abstracts.
14 Central Statistical Office (1989). op. cit.
15 Central Statistical Office (1989). op. cit.
16 Cited by Morris, J. (1988). op. cit.
17 Central Statistical Office (1989). op. cit.
18 Conway, J. (ed.) (1988). *Prescription for Poor Health: The Crisis for Homeless Families*. London Food Commission; Maternity Alliance; SHAC; Shelter.
19 Byrne, D., Harrisson, S., Keithley, J. *et al.* (1986). *Housing and Health: The Relationship between Housing Conditions and the Health of Council Tenants*. Aldershot, Gower.
20 Kemp, P. (1989). op. cit.
21 SHAC (1988). *Caught in the Act: A Critical Guide to the 1988 Housing Act*. London, SHAC.
22 Department of the Environment (1986). *English House Condition Survey*. London, HMSO.
23 Department of the Environment (1985). *An Enquiry into the Condition of Local Authority Housing Stock in England*. London, HMSO.
24 Brown, C. (1984). *Black and White Britain*. Third PSI Survey. London, Heinemann Educational.
25 Department of the Environment (1986). op. cit.
26 Luthera, M. (1989). op. cit.

27 Commission for Racial Equality (1984a). *Race and Council Housing in Hackney.* London, Commission for Racial Equality.
28 Commission for Racial Equality (1984b). *Race and Housing in Liverpool: A Research Report.* London, Commission for Racial Equality.
29 Luthera, M. (1989). op. cit.
30 Morris, J. (1988). op. cit.
31 Brook, J. (1990). *Housing Research and Policy, Conference Paper, Making Housing Fit the Facts.* The Royal Institute of Public Health, 29 January.
32 Morris, J. (1988). op. cit.
33 Central Statistical Office (1989). *Social Trends,* no. 19. London, HMSO.
34 Berthoud, R. and Kempson, E. (1990). *Credit and Debt in Britain.* London, Policy Studies Institute.
35 Berthoud, R. (1989). *Credit, Debt and Poverty,* Research Paper no. 1, Social Security Advisory Committee. London, HMSO.
36 Graham, H. (1987). 'Women's poverty and caring', in Glendinning, C. and Millar, J. (eds) *Women and Poverty in Britain.* Brighton, Wheatsheaf.
37 Berthoud, R. (1989). op. cit.
38 Kogevinas, E. (1990). *1971–1983 England and Wales: Longitudinal Study: Socio-demographic Differences in Cancer Survival.* London, HMSO.
39 Platt, S., Martin, C., Hunt, J. *et al.* (1989). 'Damp housing, mould growth and symptomatic health status' *British Medical Journal,* vol. 208, 24 June: 1673–8.
40 Brennan, M. and Lancashire, R. (1978). 'Association of childhood mortality with housing status and unemployment' *Journal of Epidemiology and Child Health,* vol. 32: 28–33.
41 Brown, G. and Harris, T. (1978). *The Social Origins of Depression: A Study of Psychiatric Disorder in Women.* London, Tavistock.
42 Gabe, J. and Williams, P. (1986). 'Is space bad for your health? The relationship between crowding in the home and the emotional distress in women' *Sociology of Health and Illness,* vol. 8, part 4: 351–71.
43 Fanning, D. (1967). 'Families in flats' *British Medical Journal,* 4: 383–6.
44 Department of the Environment (1981). *Families in Flats.* London, HMSO.
45 Department of the Environment (1986). op. cit.
46 Littlewood, J. and Tinker, A. (1981). op. cit.
47 Gittus, E. (1976). *Flats, Families, and the Under Fives.* London, Routledge & Kegan Paul.
48 Coleman, A. (1985). *Utopia on Trial: Vision and Reality in Planned Housing.* London, Hilary Shipman.
49 Glendinning, C. (1986). *A Single Door.* London, Allen & Unwin.
50 Child Accident Prevention Trust (1986). *Child Safety and Housing.* London, Bedford Square Press/NVCO.
51 Byrne, D. *et al.* (1986). op. cit.
52 Townsend, P. (1979). *Poverty in the United Kingdom.* London, Penguin.
53 Department of the Environment (1981). *Families in Flats.* London, HMSO.
54 Darley, C. (1981). 'High density housing: the Wirral's experience' *Royal Society of Health Journal,* 101, 6: 229–33.
55 Department of the Environment (1986). Cited by Drennan V. and Stearn, J., 'Health visitors and homeless families' *Health Visitor Journal,* November, vol. 59: 340–2.
56 Conway, J. (ed.) (1988). op. cit.

57 Stearn, J. (1986). 'An expensive way of making children ill' *Roof*, September/
    October: 12–14.
58 Cited by Stearn, J. (1986). *ibid*.
59 Conway, J. (ed.) (1988). op. cit.

5 | PARENTS: STRESS, COPING AND HEALTH BEHAVIOUR

INTRODUCTION

In the previous chapters we have seen how some dimensions of poverty – poor access to healthy food and fuel, poor housing conditions, and homelessness – affect health. The comments of families who experience these living conditions alert us to the fact that, above all, poverty is a daily struggle that permeates the whole of family life. This personal experience of coping with poverty is, itself, worthy of examination. For not only does it increase our knowledge of what poverty means for families, it also deepens our understanding of how living on low income affects mental well-being. Studies suggest that across the spectrum of feelings associated with mental distress, from feelings of malaise through to symptoms of mental illness, it is people in low-income groups who suffer most.

The study of the relationship between poverty and mental well-being is important for another reason: it helps us to see how mental-health status plays a part in shaping health behaviour. Research studies indicate that higher levels of unhealthy behaviours among low-income groups can be partly explained in terms of the role they play in protecting mental health. Certain behaviours, such as cigarette smoking and certain child-rearing practices, appear to help parents cope with the stress of low-income living, whilst at the same time undermining physical health.

Personal health and financial status both have moral connotations attached to them. Those who are unhealthy and those who are poor are often the same group and can find themselves reproached and held personally responsible for their poor health and social conditions. As health and welfare interventions and policy options depend on views about the causes of these problems, those who see the health and social problems of the poor in terms of 'weakness' and inability to manage their resources effectively will ascribe different solutions from those who see the coping behaviour and health of the poor as the outcome of not only social and economic deprivation, but also the stress and sense of frustration and oppression that accompanies these conditions. Competing claims needs to be addressed through research that seeks to gain a better understanding of the psychosocial implications of relative poverty.

For health and welfare fieldworkers a key question to be answered is 'How does the stress and daily struggle associated with living in poverty affect the health and behaviour of families?' This chapter will examine this key question in relation to the mental health and behaviour of parents. It will cover the following areas:

- *Patterns of mental health problems among parents:* paying attention to the influence of family structure, gender and 'race', income and employment on mental-health patterns.
- *The relationship between poverty and mental health:* drawing together the research on stress and depression together with what we know about the experience of parenting in poverty.
- *Coping strategies in poverty:* here the chapter will briefly examine two health behaviours that are commonly associated with stress – alcohol use and cigarette smoking.

The lack of research data on the links between poverty and mental health means that interpretations must be tentative. None the less, because of the importance of the issues concerned, this chapter, while exploring the links between poverty and mental health, will move beyond the limited data and suggest ways in which these links can be understood. As much of the research data relates to women, this chapter will inevitably concentrate on women's experiences. Although this fails to recognize the experience of men as parents, the fact that women remain the principal carers of children and managers of household resources justifies this focus on women.

PATTERNS OF MENTAL HEALTH
AND ILLNESS

Before we move on to examine the relationship between mental health and poverty, it is useful to identify what we mean by the term 'mental health'. The term implies more than the absence of mental-illness symptoms and generally includes the subjective feelings of mental well-being, feelings of self-worth and self-esteem, and the ability to carry out social and emotional roles and relationships. These dimensions of mental health are important to study: the experience of poverty is likely to lead to feelings of mental distress and malaise. And whilst these feelings may go on to cause mental illness in some individuals, in others they affect an individual's quality of life and sense of well-being without necessarily causing mental-illness symptoms. In any study of poverty and health, forms of mental distress are as important to study as mental illness.

Indicators of mental health are poor in comparison to indicators of mental illness. Whilst we can look at some studies that have examined the relationship between components of mental health such as social integration, the relationship between mental-health status and poverty remains an underresearched field. Lack of direct data on mental health and income means that, inevitably, we are forced to rely on mental-illness data. If we examine patterns of mental illness/mental health it is clear that there are significant differences between social groups: between high- and low-income groups, men and women, Black and white people, employed people and unemployed people, and people in different family structures. These dimensions will be examined in the next five sub-sections.

INCOME AND MENTAL HEALTH

A number of studies have examined the relationship between social class and mental health, documenting a positive link between high social class and good mental health.[1,2] In comparison, there has been little research which has examined the relationship between income and mental health. As we have seen in previous chapters, income is a key resource that determines access to vital physical resources for health. Income also determines access to emotional resources: to social support networks, to power structures and participation in social events. Money brings with it high social status. It brings choice and influence to solve problems and buys domestic comfort. Clearly we need to examine whether the stress and sense of frustration of being denied access to these resources affects mental health.

The most useful information on income and mental health comes from the *Health and Lifestyles Survey*.[3] This survey examined how various dimensions of health, including psycho-social health (which broadly equates to the view of mental health used in this book), are related to a number of socio-economic circumstances, individual characteristics, attitudes, beliefs and behaviour. Data from this survey indicated that at all ages, both men and women living in low-income households had poorer psychosocial health (and physical health) than the average population. Moreover, the data suggested that low income (independent of social class) increased the likelihood of poor psycho-social health.

Other studies, while focusing on how aspects of people's lives (usually women's lives) are linked to mental illness, have highlighted how financial stress, and dimensions of low income are linked to depression:

 Richman, Stevenson and Graham (1982) found high rates of depression among women with children, and that factors such as money worries and poor housing appeared to fuel depression.[4]

TABLE 5.1   All admissions to hospitals and units for selected mental illnesses, 1986

Diagnosis	Male	Female
Affective psychoses	8,107	16,526
Depressive disorders	11,740	23,469
Neurotic disorders	4,978	10,291
Alcohol problems	10,905	4,978
Drug dependency	1,382	806
All diagnoses	83,865 (42%)	113,386 (58%)

Source: Department of Health (1988). *Health and Personal Social Service Statistics for England, 1986*. London, HMSO

Data from the *Health and Lifestyles Survey* and studies of mental health indicate that the relationship between income and mental health is not straightforward. Other factors such as gender, race, household structure, employment status and levels of social integration interlink with income to determine the mental-health status of individuals.

GENDER AND MENTAL HEALTH

Patterns of mental health are highly related to gender. *Research into rates of mental illness inform us that women in most ethnic groups are more likely than men to be diagnosed as mentally ill in Britain.* Data on admission rates indicate that significantly more women than men are admitted to psychiatric hospitals and units. In 1986, women accounted for 58 per cent of all admissions to psychiatric hospitals and units, whilst men made up 42 per cent.[5] (see table 5.1). From the data on admission rates, it appears that women are admitted with different types of mental-illness diagnoses from men. Women are more likely to be admitted to hospital with diagnoses of affective psychoses and neurotic and depressive disorders, whilst men are more likely to be admitted with alcohol-related and drug-dependency problems (see table 5.1). Prevalence estimates from representative community studies indicate higher depression rates among women, with 12–17 per cent of women estimated as suffering from depression compared to only 6 per cent of men.[6]

Patterns of psychiatric drug use are used as a further indicator of mental ill health. Tranquillizer use appears to have a gender-specific pattern of prescription and use. The evidence suggests that women are more likely to be on tranquillizers than men. A survey of tranquillizer use in 1984 indicated that 23 per cent of the population had used tranquillizers at some time in their life. Of those who had used them women were two times more likely to use them than men.[7] The main users of tranquillizers appear to be housewives and unemployed and older adults. The peak ages for prescribed tranquillizers for women are what are generally the child-caring years (age 25–35) and the years when children are generally leaving home (age 45–54 years).[8] Very little is known about the use of tranquillizers among women from minority ethnic groups, particularly Asian women.

There is some debate about the meaning of gender differences in the rates of mental illness. On the one hand it is suggested that they may simply reflect the increased tendency of health and welfare workers to label women's symptoms as mental illness. For example, symptoms that may be labelled as overwork in men may be labelled as depression and inability to cope in women. There is also evidence that indicates that higher mental-illness rates amongst women reflect women's increased willingness to report symptoms.[9] Studies have also indicated that women and men express their stress in gender-specific ways. Whereas men are more likely to turn to alcohol, drug abuse and violent crime, women are more likely to express their feelings in more silent and self-effacing ways, hence their higher incidence of depression-type symptoms and tranquillizer use. An alternative explanation is that higher rates of mental illness may indicate women's susceptibility to mental illness. Indeed, many studies do highlight the fact that certain aspects of women's lives and social environment (particularly their role as carers and managers of household resources) can have a negative effect on mental health.[10] For these women the risk of mental illness appears to increase in the presence of adverse social and economic circumstances. Some of these factors will be examined later in this chapter.

'RACE' AND MENTAL HEALTH

Another important influence on patterns of mental health and mental illness in Britain is 'race' and ethnicity. First, like white groups, Black and minority ethnic groups suffer emotionally (as well as materially) from the experience of poverty. However, unlike white groups, they experience an additional stress that arises from the daily experience of racial discrimination. Second, there is evidence that racism within psychiatry influences the assessment, diagnosis and treatment of mental-health problems in Black and minority groups.

Although there is a relative paucity of official information on the mental-health patterns of minority ethnic groups, the evidence from individual studies indicates that ethnicity, particularly the experience of being Black, has a strong influence on mental health. Unfortunately most of the information that does exist is limited by the way the statistics are collected. In almost all studies ethnicity is inferred from information about the person's country of birth: we know very little about the health of individuals from ethnic minority groups who were born in the United Kingdom and make up a significant part of the community. Moreover, research has concentrated on mental-illness symptoms that interest doctors – schizophrenia and other psychotic illnesses – rather than the subjective experiences of minority ethnic groups themselves. Several studies have analysed data by country of birth, providing information that relates to the number and characteristics of admissions to psychiatric hospitals, types of diagnoses and the type of treatment prescribed.

These studies indicate that people born outside the UK have higher admission rates to psychiatric hospitals than UK-born adults:

 People born in Afro-Caribbean countries have higher admission rates to psychiatric hospitals than UK-born adults.[11]

 Some studies show that Asian people born outside the UK have higher admission rates to psychiatric hospitals than UK-born adults,[12] but others show mixed results.[13]

Polish, Scottish and Irish immigrants have been found to have higher admission rates to psychiatric hospitals than people born in England and Wales.[14]

However, evidence that rests solely on hospital admission rates is limited. A number of factors appear to affect the likelihood of someone's being admitted to hospital. These include factors such as availability of beds, referral practices, cultural attitudes, availability of other forms of treatment, as well as the type of symptoms exhibited by the patient.

Data on diagnoses and treatment patterns indicate that Black people born outside the UK are over-represented at the psychotic end of the diagnostic spectrum:

Cochrane (1977) found that West Indians were more likely to be diagnosed as schizophrenic than any other group.[15]

Some commentators have identified the apparent ease with which Black people can acquire labels such as 'mentally ill' or 'schizophrenic'. Researchers have pointed out that Black people may be diagnosed as schizophrenic or mentally ill, even though their symptoms may be atypical of schizophrenia or other types of mental illness.[16] This suggests that biases affect the diagnosing patterns of psychiatrists. Over-representation of Black people at the psychotic end of the spectrum has been explained in terms of the failure of psychiatrists to understand the cultural behaviour of patients.[17] It is suggested that failure to understand the cultural background of Black and minority ethnic groups has led to inappropriate diagnoses of mental illness.[18] Behaviour that is acceptable in one culture tends to be viewed as 'abnormal' in another. Torkington (1983)[19] suggests that 'cultural racism' influences diagnosing and treatment patterns; the problem arises when the white culture is assumed to be superior, and other cultures are perceived and treated as deviant and bizarre to the extent of labelling those who belong to them as psychotic or schizophrenic. Littlewood and Lipsedge (1982)[20] found evidence of biases. When a standardized interview technique was used, many patients who had previously been given the dignoses of schizophrenia could be classified as having short-lasting psychotic reactions rather than schizophrenia.

Whilst Black people tend to be over-represented at the psychotic end of the spectrum, they are under-represented at the depressive end of the spectrum. This may be explained in terms of the failure of psychiatrists to recognize symptoms of depression in Black people. Studies of depressed patients attending psychiatric services have found that Asian men reported symptoms including sexual impotency, and Asian women headaches, a 'spinning head' or sleeplessness. West Indian men complain of loss of strength and inability to work, and West Indian women infertility and headaches.[21]

Cultural racism within psychiatry also appears to ensure that, once in contact with the psychiatric services, Black people are more likely to be involuntarily detained in hospital than white people.[22] They also receive more physical treatments, such as electroconvulsive therapy, and receive more powerful drugs, particularly major tranquillizers and are less likely to receive psychotherapy than UK-born adults with similar diagnoses.[23]

Poor knowledge about the cultural aspects of mental health and racism within psychiatry may offer some explanation for higher rates of mental illness among immigrant groups than their UK-born counterparts. However, other factors are also likely to play a part in influencing both the physical and mental health of ethnic minority groups. The culture shock and discrimination experienced by immigrants from Third World countries may lead to feelings of alienation, social isolation and stress, which may precipitate mental illness.[24] Race-relations research on institutional and individual racism in British society offers an alternative or additional explanation. Although some immigrants may arrive in this country with poorer health in the first place, any existing health problems are compounded by the fact that, like many British-born minority groups, they are over-represented in manual occupations. They often live in poor housing, in the poorest environments, with few employment opportunities and low incomes. They suffer the health disadvantages associated with being working class – and more.[25] Furthermore, communication difficulties and health and social services that fail to take into account the needs of Britain's minority ethnic population only add to their problems. Eyles and Donovan's study (1990)[26] of lay perceptions of health and illness illustrated that, for Black people, there was a clear link between the racism they experienced daily and their health state:

It affects your mind. If you feel depressed that you are not treated as other people are or they look down on you, you will feel mentally ill, won't you? It will depress you that you are not treated as good as you would be in your own country. So if you are not treated well racially, it will affect your health in some way. It will cause depression, and the depression will cause the illness.

(Comments of an Asian woman)[27]

Few authors have investigated the effect of material deprivation and racism on the health status of minority ethnic groups. The link between the experience of individual and institutional racism and poor mental health is an area that requires further research. The need to improve the quality, and quantity of research on the mental-health patterns and experiences of both Black and minority ethnic groups born abroad and those who have been born in the UK is paramount.

HOUSEHOLD STRUCTURE AND MENTAL HEALTH

Research studies suggest family and household structure have a strong influence on the mental-health status of household members.

Mental health is related to marital status. For both men and women, being married, or having a partner, generally has a positive effect on mental health. Married or cohabiting couples appear to have better mental health than either single, divorced or separated people living without partners.[28,29]

The presence of children has also been shown to be a factor that influences the mental health of parents. The presence of children has a marked effect on the mental health of lone mothers (see table 5.2). This finding is not new and has been documented by other studies. For example, Burnell and Wadsworth's study (1981)[30] of mental-illness rates among mothers found higher rates of stress and poorer mental health among lone mothers than mothers in two-parent families. No similar work appears to have been done on the mental health of lone fathers, perhaps because they form a significantly smaller group than lone mothers and are more likely to go out to work. Whilst the *Health and Lifestyles Survey* indicated that the presence of children, in the absence of other factors, made little overall difference to the mental health of married couples or cohabiting couples (see table 5.2), both this study and other studies have indicated that the presence of children, combined with the presence or absence of other factors, can affect the mental health of mothers (there are no data on fathers). Some of these factors have been discussed in other chapters, for example, the experience of living above ground level, or in overcrowded accommodation. These studies highlight that other factors such as the experience of racism, employment status, and level of social support interlink with income and gender to determine a person's mental health status.

EMPLOYMENT STATUS AND MENTAL HEALTH

For women with children, employment status appears to have an important bearing on mental health. Gender, paid work and parenthood appear to

TABLE 5.2   Psycho-social-health ratio* for women with and without children (age-standardized)

	Psycho-social health	
	Age 18–29	Age 30–45
Lone parent	137	142
Married or cohabiting, with children	99	97
Married or cohabiting, without children	89	99

* Psycho-social-health ratio refers to the relationship of a group compared to the average for the population, with the figure 100 representing the mean. Thus a value of more than 100 means that a group has poorer psycho-social health than a group with a score below 100.
Source: Blaxter, M. (1990). Health and Lifestyles. London, Routledge

combine in a complex way to protect the mental health of some women, whilst acting to reduce the mental health of others. From an analysis of the Health and Lifestyles Survey data Blaxter[31] concludes that, for married or cohabiting women, paid employment outside the home may have no ill effect on the mental health of mothers and indeed may be beneficial if the job is pleasant and well paid and satisfactory childcare resources are available. However, if a mother works outside the home primarily because of the need to increase the household income, finds her job unpleasant and has poor childcare resources, then her mental health may suffer.

Men's employment status appears to affect both their own health and the health of their partners. Studies of the health effects of unemployment have indicated that unemployed people have higher rates of mental and physical ill health than employed people.[32,33] Other studies have found an association between unemployment and suicide and attempted suicide, with the highest rates found among those who live in areas of multiple disadvantage.[34] Moreover, studies which have documented the effect of male unemployment on family life have shown that the mental health of wives, partners and children can suffer.[35]

It has been argued that high rates of mental and physical ill health among unemployed people may reflect a situation where those with poor health are most likely to become unemployed. However, while this is likely to account for some of the findings, it cannot explain the excess of mental and physical ill health found among unemployed people. A more plausible explanation is that unemployment affects the health of individuals through stress and the effect of low income.

THE RELATIONSHIP BETWEEN POVERTY AND MENTAL HEALTH

From an examination of the patterns of mental health, it appears that those social groups who suffer the poorest mental health – women, particularly women with children, unemployed people and Black people – are also the groups who commonly find themselves in poverty. Whilst patterns of mental illness indicate a positive association between poverty and poor mental health, they do not necessarily indicate the nature of the relationship. This prompts us to ask the question 'Do the social and economic circumstances associated with poverty influence a person's mental-health status in some way or is there a process of social selection at work, where those with poor mental health drift down the social scale into poverty?' Research indicates that a two-way process is at work. There is little doubt that individuals with poor mental health are at higher risk of poverty than those with good mental health. Employment, housing, social-security and community-care policies are ill equipped to provide adequate support and resources for people with mental-health problems. Like physical illness, a long-term mental illness reduces an individual's ability to find or maintain employment, thereby increasing reliance on social-security benefits and reducing access to other health resources. The social-security system is not designed to cope with mental ill health which tends to fluctuate in its duration and severity. Social-security regulations are complicated concerning therapeutic earnings, earnings disregard and fitness for work. They often fail to meet the needs of people with mental ill health. And whilst community-care grants from the social fund are designed to give increased resources to people who are being discharged from long-stay institutions under 'care in the community' policies, many commentators have argued that they are inadequate and do not provide for the majority of people with mental-health problems who are already cared for at home.[36]

Although the higher risk of poverty among people with poor mental health explains some of the association between increased rates of mental illness and poverty, it cannot entirely account for it. Neither can arguments that derive from the medical model of mental illness and try to explain mental-illness symptoms as the manifestation of some underlying personality deficit account for this association. Research studies that have tried to explain the greater vulnerability of some social groups have highlighted that a person's social and economic environment influences his or her mental health status. These studies suggest that factors including income, the presence of children, employment status, gender and 'race' interact together in a complex way to determine a person's exposure to stress and ability to mitigate the effects of that stress.

The comments of poor families indicate that feelings of stress and powerlessness feature strongly in their daily experience of poverty. Living on low income allows little scope to cope with the day-in, day-out pressures of limited access to material resources. Research that has sought to identify the determinants of mental health have drawn attention to the way psychological factors – from life-events, poor social integration (a low level of social ties with others) and low levels of social support – influence health and behaviour. In the next three sub-sections the chapter will look at the relationship between stress and mental illness, the contribution of confiding relationships and social support to mental health and, last, the link between stress and parenting in poor living conditions.

STRESS AND MENTAL HEALTH

A belief in a link between stress and ill health is not new. Eyles and Donovan's study (1990) found that almost all respondents identified worry as a significant cause of illness: 'So many illnesses come on because of the worries. Tension, mental tension – you can't sleep very well with the tension. Then when that will pass, it will lead to illness, won't it?' (an Asian woman).[37]

This lay belief has been repeatedly confirmed by research that has sought to examine the nature of the link between stress and ill health. To examine the link between poverty and mental health we need to understand the role of stress in mental ill health. Stress is an everyday part of all our lives and does not necessarily lead to pathological changes. At low levels it acts as a stimulus to achieve goals and progress and improves performance. However, too much stress or inadequate coping resources can cause ill health. Specific forms of stress appear to be associated with certain kinds of mental and physical illness: depression, anxiety problems, heart disease, gastro-intestinal diseases and lowered immunity to infections.[38,39]

Much of our present knowledge about the role of stress in mental illness comes from studies that have examined rates of depression among women. This work has pointed to a link between life-events and depression. Statistical pooling of data suggests that stressful life events make a significant total contribution to mental illness, particularly depression.[40] Studies of the role of life-events in depression indicate that it is the *meaning* of life-events to individuals rather than change itself that is important.[41,42] One of the most useful pieces of UK research on the role of life-events in mental illness is Brown and Harris's study (1978)[43] of the social origins of depression in women.

This study indicated that the key provoking agents for depression were not just any life-events, but life-events that signified long-term social loss or threat. For example, actual separation or threat of separation from a key person through death or serious illness, major material loss, loss of employment or failure to attain major personal goals were all associated with an increased risk of depression. Changes to routine or social contacts or short-term threats are rarely enough to cause depression, unless they serve to bring home the implications of some on-going major loss or disappointment.

Brown and Harris's study recorded significantly higher rates of depression amongst working-class women with children than amongst comparable middle-class women. Working-class women with children at home had a four-fold greater risk of developing depression than comparable middle-class women. There was no class difference in the risk of depression among women without children. The highest rate of depression was found among working-class women with a child under six years old at home. This prompted the researchers to ask 'What is it about the lives of working-class women with children that increases their risk of depression?' Researchers have identified both the material conditions of people's lives and a number of vulnerability factors, some of which are closely linked to people's social and economic position, as factors that influence mental health.

Several research studies have found an association between the stress associated with poverty and poor mental health. Brown and Harris's study found that a significant number of working-class women lived in adverse social conditions, and suffered more severe life-events and difficulties involving social loss than middle-class women.[44] For these women, low income is likely to determine their social-class experience. Material loss and social loss have greater implications for low-income families than higher-income families, particularly women in low-income families. As we have seen in previous chapters, women are at the sharp end of poverty and social adversity. Women bear the brunt of poverty. Moreover, as gate-keepers of family health, women frequently experience the worry and stress of budgeting to make ends meet and managing debts. For families with higher incomes, good living conditions and adequate income can cushion the effect of social loss. For example, for low-income families, the worries associated with finding the money to cover funeral costs are likely to compound feelings of grief when a loved one dies. Other studies have also found an association between poverty and mental-health problems. Financial poverty, debt problems, difficulty meeting bills and poor housing have all been strongly associated with depression:

> Richman, Stevenson and Graham's study (1982) of families with pre-school children in Waltham Forest identified high rates of mental-health problems among mothers, and that these were strongly related to poor housing conditions, unemployment and money worries.[45]

Poverty itself is likely to bring about more severe life-events: bereavement, loss of employment, threat of loss due to serious illness or accidents for families. This greater adversity and higher risk of severe life-events explains partly, but not wholly, the higher risk of depression and mental illness among low-income groups.

Researchers have identified a number of vulnerability factors that mediate between stressful life-events and depression, by influencing a person's ability to cope effectively with social loss. The most commonly identified factors include the lack of a confiding relationship, the presence of young children, social isolation, lack of self-esteem and feelings of lack of control.[46,47]

It is probable that a large part of social-class differences in rates of depression stems from the fact that factors that appear to militate against the successful resolution of stress occur more frequently among low-income groups than high-income groups. Most of the social-class differences in rates of depression in Brown and Harris's study can be explained by the fact that working-class women had more vulnerability factors than other women.[48] These vulnerability factors, with the exception of having lost one's own mother before the age of eleven years, are linked to a person's social and economic position.

Fisher[49] has suggested a further mechanism by which stress may influence mental health. Fisher's theory of locus of control suggests that a person who feels in control of events may be able to cope with stress more effectively, thus avoiding stress-related illness, than a person who does not feel in control. A person's perception of control over events depends on a number of factors, including personality factors, previous experience and the nature of the current situation. Fisher suggests that social and economic deprivation may weaken a person's belief that he or she can exercise control. The frequent experience of reduced control leads to further feelings that control is rarely possible in life and pessimism about personal ability to solve problems.

> Poverty curtails freedom of choice. The freedom to eat as you wish, to go where and when you like, to seek the leisure pursuits or political activities which others accept; all are denied to those without the resources . . .[50]

CONFIDING RELATIONSHIPS AND SOCIAL SUPPORT

A confiding relationship with a partner and social support from family members, friends, and neighbours have been shown to be important determinants of good mental health. Good relationships with partners, relatives, and friends appear to protect against the negative effects of stressful life-events by increasing feelings of self-worth and offering emotional and practical support. Those who have low levels of social integration appear to have poorer mental health than those who are highly socially integrated:

 Blaxter (1990) identified poorer psycho-social health among people with low social integration scores.[51]

 Brown and Harris (1978) found high rates of depression among women without confiding relationships.[52]

Higher rates of poor mental health among low-income groups may be partly explained by lower levels of social integration and social support among low-income groups than among higher-income groups.

The contribution of a confiding relationship to mental health is likely to explain, at least in part, why people with partners have better mental health than single, separated or divorced people. The fact that Brown and Harris found that working-class women were less likely to have a confiding relationship than other women can partly be explained in terms of their social and economic position. For example, the majority of lone mothers fall into low-income groups, or the category working class. Poor access to training, and secure and well-paid jobs, and the difficulty of finding satisfactory and affordable childcare facilities militate against lone mothers moving into higher-income or middle-class occupations. Being a lone mother with dependent children restricts opportunities to socialize, to meet new partners or meet new people through paid work.

Four main influences appear to determine the levels and type of social support people receive: social position, gender, 'race' and life stage:

Social integration and support from family and friends appears to be strongly class related. Middle-class people tend to have larger networks of friends than working-class people, but working-class people make up for fewer friends by seeing them more often. Working-class people tend to see more of relatives than middle-class people.[53] Willmot has suggested that social-class differences in patterns of social support result from differences in access to material resources and social-class tradition. In his study of friendship and social support networks,[54] he found that on every index, social status and affluence went with larger social networks. First, material resources determine which families can afford to entertain and meet friends, and who has the housing conditions to entertain friends at home. Car ownership appears to affect opportunities for sociable mixing crucially, hence the number of friends and their spread and diversity. Being able to afford telephones and bus or train fares, to travel to visit friends and families also help individuals to receive support from important people in their lives. Second, tradition affects styles of friendship and support. Whilst middle-class styles of friendship are becoming more common among working-class people, working-class people continue to see friends somewhere other than inside the home.

Patterns of social integration and types of networks differ with gender. Men and women have equally large social networks. Women's networks tend to be more home and locally based, particularly for mothers with dependent children. Gender segregation of friends is commoner among working-class people.[55] Gender differences in social-support patterns appear to be related to gender roles. For example, women with children tend to have home-based and local social contact networks, whereas men tend to have networks based outside the home.

Patterns of social support differ between ethnic groups. Extensive support may be available from extended families or from the religious or the social community for some ethnic groups, for example, well-established Jewish, Asian, Chinese, Afro-Caribbean and Irish communities. For people who have newly moved from their own country, and for those who live away from members of the same ethnic groups, separation can lead to feelings of emotional and social isolation, and lack of practical help. Mayall and Foster's study of mothers in London found that mothers who had been in the UK less than ten years felt the lack of mothers and sisters. Migration had cut them off from sources of advice and support. Phoning relatives abroad was an important item to budget for in many families.[56]

Families and individuals have different levels of social integration and support at different life-stages. Families with dependent children, older adults and people with disabilities have high social-support needs.[57] Support from their family, friends and neighbours can have a protective effect on mental health. Social support can reduce the effects of stresses that appear to be an inherent part of bringing up children. Studies of social-support networks indicate that relatives (particularly parents and parents-in-law) appear to be the main source of social support at times of children's illnesses, with baby sitting and with financial problems and loans:

> I think having somebody close to you is very important. There were a couple of times when I just dumped Peter on my mum and said, 'You have him, because if I have him he's just going in the bin!'
>
> (Mother of child under one year)[58]

Friends (particularly neighbours) are also important sources of social support, especially if a family has no relatives living nearby. Friends offer day-to-day help, act as confidantes, provide sociability and are often valued for the empathy that comes from shared experiences. Having contact and help from someone who shares similar experiences has been shown to be a very valuable form of social support, particularly for mothers with young dependent children:

> She'll [friend] give me little tips and I'll give her little tips . . . I see her every Wednesday. At this age, differences in three months are really dramatic. All little different things I'd seen her baby do I'd see him [her own baby] doing.
>
> (Mother with young baby)[59]

However, low-income families have little choice about where they live (see chapter 4); thus they may find themselves housed away from their main support networks. This is particularly the case for families who have newly arrived from abroad, or families in temporary accommodation. Public and private housing policies often fail to recognize the importance of placing vulnerable groups, such as families with young children, older adults and families with people with disabilities near their family and friends. Furthermore, housing design, particularly multi-storey block design, appears to actively work against socialization and interaction with neighbours. Townsend's concept of 'environmental poverty' (see chapter 4) also alerts us to the fact that many low-income families are housed in areas that have few community resources. Playgroups, community centres, community groups and social and recreational facilities serve to promote social-support networks by putting people in touch with each other.

McKee's study (1987)[60] of how families with young children 'get by' during unemployment indicates that giving and receiving support from family and friends is not always as harmonious or straightforward as implied by other studies. Acts of support and generosity do not always lead to feelings of appreciation and can cause feelings of resentment and conflict. McKee suggests that informal support cannot be separated off from wider cultural assumptions about social roles and obligations. Whilst it is commonly accepted that help is offered and received at times of natural disasters and major transitions, such as the birth of a child, or bereavement, the rules governing help in times of unemployment or unremitting poverty are much more muddled.

Willmot's study indicated that only a minority of families (approximately 5–10 per cent) received very little help, and these families are most likely to be in poor social and economic circumstances.[61] Low-income families not only face more barriers to receiving support than other families, they are also likely to face more barriers to giving material and social help than higher-income households. McKee's study and other studies[62] indicate that low-income households are less likely to have the material resources to offer service exchanges or help.

STRESS, PARENTING AND POOR LIVING CONDITIONS

Several research studies[63,64] have identified that being a parent increases the risk of depression, especially for women. This risk appears to rise with the presence of young children, and with increasing numbers of children. It is highest for women with three or more children under fourteen years, with at least one under six years. What is it about the lives of women with dependent children that increases their risk of depression? Brown and Harris's study supports other research data indicating that women's position in the social structure and their role and responsibilities as parents make their lives inherently more stressful and depressing.

First, caring for young children at home can be stressful in itself. In Graham's study of the organization of family health care (1986), 90 per cent of mothers said they found childcare stressful at times.[65] For many women, caring for children at home is a twenty-four-hour physically and emotionally demanding job, with no pay, low status and poor work conditions. Whilst certain aspects of caring for children are common to all mothers, the conditions under which mothers care vary with income, and the research evidence suggests that conditions are poorest and most stressful for mothers in low-income families (see chapters 3 and 4). Chapter 6 will examine how a lack of health resources and the stress of parenting in poverty affect childcare practices.

Second, caring for children can be socially isolating. Graham's study of mothers with young children found that between one-quarter to one-third of mothers said they were lonely.[66] Many women with children find it difficult to maintain old networks of friends. Limited access to training, and well-paid and secure jobs, together with the problem of finding affordable and satisfactory childcare facilities, prevents mothers from experiencing contact with others and the rewards of going out to work. This is particularly likely to be the case for lone mothers. The conditions under which many low-income mothers live also make it difficult to get out to meet others.

The stress of parenting in poverty has also been associated with higher rates of child abuse. It has been suggested that it is appropriate to see child abuse as the result of multiple interacting factors, including the family's place in the social structure, the balance of external support and stresses and the psychological traits of parents and children.[67] Several researchers have suggested that low income, combined with disruptive demographic factors and poor external social support, generate the stress and life crises that place children at risk and may precipitate child abuse.[68,69] This work indicates that child-protection work needs to be placed in the context of the debate about child care: that is, the way society cares for children and, in particular, the resources available to individuals and communities for childcare. Garbarino's work on the differences between neighbourhoods with high and low risks of child abuse has indicated that, in areas of social and economic disadvantage, the availability of mutual social support and help within the neighbourhood can reduce the neighbourhood risk of child abuse. Garbarino found that where families with high social-support needs were clustered together, families were less likely to be able to offer each other mutual aid or support. Child abuse rates were higher in these areas. Rates of child abuse appear to be higher among low-income families. However, this can be partially explained by the fact that low-income families, particularly lone-parent families, are often subjected to higher rates of surveillance than high-income families. Child abuse also occurs in better-off families but it is less likely to be identified.

Whilst the data suggest that the stress of parenting in poverty may be a factor in child abuse, to indicate in any way that low-income families are at high risk of abusing their children would be wrong. Clearly, the majority of children in poor families are loved and cared for well. In the following chapter, how well families care in the face of adversity will be discussed.

COPING AND HEALTH BEHAVIOUR: SMOKING AND ALCOHOL USE

The stress of living on low income not only affects how parents care for their children's health, it also appears to shape how parents care for their own health. Alcohol, tobacco and drug use and food behaviours are commonly brought to our attention by those in the health-promotion and health-policy field as aspects of lifestyle that are closely linked to the killer diseases of the

TABLE 5.3   Average weekly household expenditure on alcohol and cigarettes, 1988, for household with two adults and two children

Gross normal weekly household income	Average weekly spending	
	Alcohol	Cigarettes
under £200	£5.93	£6.35
£200–£299	£8.64	£5.77
£300–£450	£10.23	£4.49
£450 plus	£13.56	£2.97

Source: Department of Employment (1990). Family Expenditure Survey, 1988. London, HMSO

late twentieth century. Moreover, they are behaviours that are often blamed on the domestic or personal incompetence of low-income families. Throughout this book it has been apparent that particular ways in which low-income parents behave can serve as coping strategies that help them to deal with, and survive, the stresses and financial hardships of family life in poverty. These behaviours, while acting to sustain coping, and probably mental health, are often health damaging. By enabling parents to cope, they appear to promote family welfare; but only by undermining individual health.[70] Several strategies have been illustrated in other chapters of this book. For example, chapter 3 illustrated how giving children food they prefer and using crisps, biscuits and sweets at strategic times helps to keep family life calm. Earlier in this chapter, it was evident that tranquillizers play a crucial role in the lives of many women, helping them to cope with the most difficult social role and the adversity of circumstances. This section will examine how two more health behaviours, alcohol use and cigarette smoking, are related to low-income living.

ALCOHOL USE AND LOW INCOME

Patterns of alcohol use are linked to ethnicity and culture. Alcohol appears to be an integral part of British culture, with over 90 per cent of British people consuming alcohol. We know less about alcohol-consumption patterns among minority ethnic groups but, as alcohol is less culturally accepted in some groups, for example, among some Asian groups, consumption patterns are likely to reflect the acceptability of alcohol within different cultures.

Patterns of alcohol use are highly linked to household income. However, unlike patterns of smoking behaviour and unhealthy food consumption, alcohol consumption and expenditure appear to be lower among low-income families than higher-income families. Table 5.3 shows patterns of household expenditure on alcohol and cigarettes. This table indicates that alcohol expenditure rises with income. Women drink less than men, with young women, with young, dependent children, having the lowest consumption rates. The belief that low-income families squander their money away on alcohol appears to be a misconception.

CIGARETTE SMOKING AND LOW INCOME

Unlike alcohol behaviour, smoking behaviour appears to be commoner amongst low-income groups. This paradox has been the source of much debate among researchers and health workers, with the result that those who are the most socially disadvantaged have frequently been the target of anti-smoking strategies. The fact that health-education campaigns seem to have little effect on those in low social groups has caused increasing confusion.

Patterns of cigarette consumption and expenditure appear to be linked to social class and income. The proportion of women smokers in manual households is nearly twice as high as the proportion found among women in the highest social group, and the pattern is similar for men, with just over two times as many men in manual households smoking as men in the highest social group.[71] Social disparities in smoking patterns are increasing, with cigarette smoking fast becoming a habit that is sustained by those in working-class households.

Cigarette smoking is closely linked to gender and ethnicity. Men smoke more than women, but smoking rates among women are failing to fall as fast as among men. This appears to be due to sharp increases in smoking among young women aged 11–16 years,[72] and the fact that women seem to find it harder to give up smoking than men.[73] Whilst smoking rates are high among women in manual classes, smoking among women in the UK is a habit practised by white women rather than Black women.[74] Divorced, separated and widowed women are more likely to smoke than women who have a male partner, or single women.[75]

Changing patterns of smoking behaviour have acted as a stimulus to researchers to examine what it is that underlies these changes. It appears that differences in smoking behaviour between groups of women cannot be explained in terms of differences in health knowledge or perceptions of financial risk. Women smokers appear to be well aware of the health and financial costs of smoking. For example, Blaxter found that 79 per cent of women smokers aged 18–39 thought that smoking was a health risk of high or medium importance.[76] Graham suggests that women's smoking is linked to their everyday experiences, particularly their experience of poverty. Smoking appears to have a crucial role in the lives of mothers. It appears to help them to cope with the psychological stress and financial hardship of bringing up children in poverty.[77] Smoking also helps women on low income make economies. For example, smoking suppresses feelings of hunger.

I think smoking stops me getting so irritable. I can cope with things better. If I was economizing, I'd cut down on cigarettes but I wouldn't give up. I'd stop eating . . . Food just isn't that important to me but having a cigarette is the only thing I do just for myself.

(Lone mother)[78]

CONCLUSION AND IMPLICATIONS FOR PRACTICE

A review of patterns of mental health and mental illness indicate that those groups who are most at risk of poverty are also likely to have the poorest mental health. The chapter has illustrated how poverty can affect psychological health. It highlights how poverty increases the level of stress families are exposed to, whilst at the same time decreasing their resources to cope with this stress. Although factors such as the level of self-esteem and the ability to cope with stress are dimensions of personality, an individual's psycho-social status appears to be strongly influenced by the daily experience of low-income living. Poverty is a daily experience of financial hardship, worry, stigma and powerlessness.

Three key points emerge from this chapter. First, families in poverty are likely to experience more stressful life-events than their better-off counterparts. Financial hardship, worries about bills and debts, poor housing conditions, an unsafe environment for children, unemployment and inadequate food, clothing, and heating all bring crises to families. But families in poverty face more than stressful life-events due to material loss. Poverty brings with it emotional loss when poverty takes its toll on the health of loved ones.

Second, families in poverty are less likely than higher-income groups to experience the social conditions that promote good mental health and the resolution of stress. Poverty appears to expose people, particularly women, to factors that increase an individual's risk of depression. The social and economic circumstances of people in poverty means that it is harder for individuals to experience good support from a partner, friends or family. Moreover, low-income families, particularly lone mothers, are exposed to the stresses of parenting on low income without having any of the material and social resources to help them cope.

Third, some low-income families appear to cope with or avoid the worst elements of this distress by adopting behaviours that help them to survive. Various child-rearing practices and parental smoking in white families appear to fit into this category. The information we have on the link between these behaviours and low income explains why traditional health-education programmes that focus on imparting knowledge and changing individual behaviour have failed among low-income groups and poses new challenges for future programmes. We know little about why relatively few people from minority groups smoke, and a greater understanding would enrich our understanding of why some people never smoke.

The relationship between mental health and poverty has implications for social policy. To improve mental health, families need higher incomes and better access to material resources. Housing conditions and policies need to promote social-support networks between families and friends, rather than working against them. Families need access to community facilities, such as community centres, recreational facilities and playgroups, which will bring people together. Sadly these facilities are frequently lacking in deprived areas, compounding the isolation of families even further. The research evidence highlights the need for more research into the needs of minority ethnic groups and demands that policies and practice redress the discrimination that these families face.

The research evidence also points to the need for health and welfare workers to acknowledge in their practice, the experience of parenting in poverty. The evidence in this chapter emphasizes the urgent need for workers to take on, or extend their role in, the area of stimulating and maintaining neighbourhood social-support and self-help networks for parents. For many workers, this will be a new area of work that demands new skills, particularly the skill of listening to what parents define as their support needs. This need is greatest in relation to the support needs of minority ethnic groups and lone parents. Furthermore, it demands that workers utilize their skills and resources to extend the social-support element within their existing work, for example, by increasing the opportunities for social contact between parents in child health clinics, schools and social-service centres. For many workers this may demand a change in focus from less one-to-one work to group work. The results of work in this area indicate that this approach has positive benefits for workers and clients. Moreover, developing good social-support networks demands more than facilitating groups. For some workers it offers the challenge to 'let go' by allowing groups to develop their own identities, focus and interests. Promoting social-support networks also offers a political challenge to workers. It defines a role where workers need to co-operate with tenants' groups to argue for better community resources and sensitive policies from statutory and voluntary agencies. While social-support initiatives and policies are vitally important for the well-being of families, it is pertinent to offer a note of caution. In the present political climate, care and support by the family and community have come to represent an alternative to care by the state. Although social support is a crucial element for a cohesive society, it is hard to see it as a viable alternative to the state provision of health and welfare services.

REFERENCES

1 Goldberg, D. and Auxley, P. (1980). *Mental Illness in the Community*. London, Tavistock.
2 Cox, B. D. *et al.* (1987). *The Health and Lifestyles Survey*. London, Health Promotion Research Trust.
3 Cox, B. D. *et al.* (1987). *ibid.*
4 Richman, N., Stevenson, J. and Graham, P. (1982). *Pre-School to School. A Behavioural Study*. London, Academic Press.
5 Department of Health (1988). *Health and Personal Social Services Statistics for England, 1986*. London, HMSO.
6 Smith, A. and Jacobson, B. (eds) (1988). *The Nation's Health: A Strategy For the 1990s*. London, King's Fund.
7 Cited by Women's National Commission (1988). *Stress and Addiction Amongst Women: Report of An Ad-Hoc Working Group*.
8 Women's National Commission (1988). *ibid.*
9 Clarke, J. (1983). 'Sexism, feminism and medicalisation – a decade review of literature on gender and illness' *Sociology of Health and Illness*, 5: 62.
10 Richman, N. *et al.* (1982). op. cit.
11 Dean, G., Walsh, D., Downing, H. *et al.* (1981). 'First admissions of native-born and immigrants to psychiatric hospitals in South-East England, 1976' *British Journal of Psychiatry*, vol. 139, 506–12.
12 Carpenter, L. and Brockington, I. (1980) 'A study of mental illness in Asians, West Indians and Africans living in Manchester' *British Journal of Psychiatry*, vol. 137, 201–5.
13 Dean, G. *et al.* (1981). op. cit.
14 Cochrane, R. (1977). Cited by Grimsley, M. and Bhat, A. (1988), chapter 7, in Bhat, A., Carr-Hill, R. and Ahri, S. (eds) (1988). *Britain's Black Population*, 2nd Edition. Aldershot, Gower.
15 Cochrane, R. (1977). Cited by Grimsley, M. and Bhat, A. (1988). *ibid.*
16 Littlewood, R. and Lipsedge, M. (1982). *Aliens and Alienists*. Harmondsworth, Penguin.
17 Donovan, J. (1984). 'Ethnicity and health: a research review' *Social Science and Medicine*, vol. 19, 7: 663–70.
18 Littlewood, R. and Lipsedge, M. (1982). op. cit.
19 Torkington, N. P. K. (1983). *The Racial Politics of Health – A Liverpool Profile*. Merseyside Area Profile Group, Dept. of Sociology, University of Liverpool.
20 Littlewood, R. and Lipsedge, M. (1982). op. cit.
21 Cited by Donovan, J. (1984). op. cit.
22 Littlewood, R. and Lipsedge, M. (1982). op. cit.
23 Littlewood, R. and Lipsedge, M. (1982). op. cit.
24 Mares, P., Henley, A. and Baxter, C. (1985). *Health Care in Multiracial Britain*. London, Health Education Council/National Extension College.
25 Grimsley, M. and Bhat, A. (1988). 'Health', in Bhat, A., Carr-Hill, R. and Ahri, S. (eds) *Britain's Black Population*, 2nd edition. Aldershot, Gower.
26 Eyles, J. and Donovan, J. (1990). *The Social Effects of Health Policy*. Aldershot, Avebury.
27 Quoted in Eyles, J. and Donovan, J. (1990). ibid.

28 Morgan, M. (1980). 'Marital status, health, illness and service use' *Social Science and Medicine*, 14A: 633–43.
29 Blaxter, M. (1990). *Health and Lifestyles*. London, Routledge.
30 Burnell, I. and Wadsworth, J. (1981). *Children in One-Parent Families*. University of Bristol.
31 Blaxter, M. (1990). op. cit.
32 Moser, K., Fox, A. and Jones, D. (1986). 'Unemployment and mortality in the Office of Populations, Censuses and Surveys' longitudinal study', in Wilkinson, E. (ed.) *Class and Health: Research and Longitudinal Data*. London, Tavistock.
33 Warr, P. (1985). 'Twelve questions about unemployment and health', in Roberts, B. *et al. New Approaches to Economic Life*. Manchester, Manchester University.
34 Kreitman, N. (1976). 'The coal gas story: UK suicide rates, 1960–1971' *British Journal of Preventive and Social Medicine*, 30, 86–93.
35 Fagan, L. and Little, L. (1984). *Forsaken Families*. Harmondsworth, Penguin.
36 Pidgeon, J. and Shepperson, G. (1988). 'Poverty and mental health', in Becker, S., MacPherson, S. (eds) *Public Issues, Private Pain*. London, Insight.
37 Quoted in Eyles, J. and Donovan, J. (1990). *The Social Effects of Health Policy*. Aldershot, Avebury.
38 Craig, T. K. and Brown, G. W. (1984). 'Goal frustration and life events in the aetiology of painful gastrointestinal disorder', cited by British Medical Association (1987). *Deprivation and Ill-Health*. British Medical Association.
39 Denman, A. M. (1986). 'Immunity and depression' *British Medical Journal*, vol. 293, 464–5.
40 Smith, A. and Jacobson, B. (1988). op. cit.
41 Brown, G. and Harris, T. (1978). *The Social Origins of Depression: A Study of Psychiatric Disorder in Women*. London, Tavistock.
42 Mechanic, D. (1962). Cited by Brown G. and Harris, T. (1978). op. cit.
43 Brown, G. and Harris, T. (1978). op. cit.
44 Brown, G. and Harris, T. (1978). op. cit.
45 Richman, N. *et al.* (1982). op. cit.
46 Brown, G. and Harris, T. (1978). op. cit.
47 Richman, N. *et al.* (1982). op. cit.
48 Brown, G. and Harris, T. (1978). op. cit.
49 Fisher, S. (1984). *Stress and the Perception of Control*. London, Lawrence Erlbaum Associates.
50 Quoted from Golding, P. (1986). *Excluding the Poor*. London, Child Poverty Action Group.
51 Blaxter, M. (1990). op. cit.
52 Brown, G. and Harris, T. (1978). op. cit.
53 Willmot, P. (1987). *Friendship Networks and Social Support*. London, Policy Studies Institute.
54 Willmot, P. (1987). *ibid.*
55 Directorate of Welsh Heart Programme (1986). *Pulse of Wales, Preliminary Report of the Welsh Heart Health Survey*, Report No. 4, Cardiff.
56 Mayall, B. and Foster, M.-C. (1990). *Child Health Care: Living with Children, Working with Children*. Oxford, Heinemann Nursing.
57 Willmot, P. (1987). op. cit.
58 Quoted in Curtice, L. (1989). *The First Year of Life*. London, Maternity Alliance.
59 Quoted in Curtice, L. (1989). *ibid.*

60 McKee, L. (1987). 'Households during unemployment: the resourcefulness of the unemployed', in Brannen, J. and Wilson, G. (eds) *Give and Take in Families*. London, Allen & Unwin.

61 Willmot, P. (1987). op. cit.

62 Pahl, R. (1984). *Divisions of Labour*. Oxford, Blackwell.

63 Brown, G. and Harris, T. (1978). op. cit.

64 Richman, N. *et al*. (1982). op. cit.

65 Graham, H. (1986). *Caring for the Family*. London, Health Education Council.

66 Graham, H. (1986). *ibid*.

67 Parton, N. (1989). 'Child abuse', in Kahan, B. (ed.) *Child Care Research, Policy and Practice*. London, Hodder & Stoughton.

68 Madge, N. (1983). 'Identifying families at risk', in Madge, N. (ed.) *Families at Risk*. London, Heinemann.

69 Garbarino, J. and Sherman, D. (1980). 'High risk neighbourhoods and high risk families: the human ecology of child maltreatment' *Child Development*, 51: 188–98.

70 Graham, H. (1984). *Women, Health and the Family*. Brighton, Wheatsheaf.

71 Office of Populations, Censuses and Surveys (1989). *The General Household Survey, 1986*. London, HMSO.

72 ASH Women and Smoking Group (1989). *Teenage Girls and Smoking*. ASH.

73 Jacobson, B. (1988). *Beating The Ladykillers*. London, Gollancz Paperbacks.

74 Marmot, M., Adelstein, A. and Bulusu, L. (1984). *Immigrant Mortality in England and Wales, 1970–78*. London, HMSO.

75 Office of Population, Census and Surveys (1989). op. cit.

76 Blaxter, M. (1990). op. cit.

77 Graham, H. (1984). op. cit.

78 Quoted by Graham, H. (1987). 'Women's poverty and caring', in Glendinning, C., Millar, J. (eds) *Women and Poverty in Britain*. Brighton, Wheatsheaf.

6 | CARING FOR CHILDREN'S HEALTH IN POVERTY

INTRODUCTION

Earlier chapters of this book have drawn attention to the fact that, as we move into the 1990s, family life and family health care for some families are set against a changing and threatening background. Over the last decade social and economic changes have adversely affected families with low incomes. The previous chapters have examined how low income exerts a major influence on the material and social environment in which parents and children live and the consequences of this for family health. This chapter is about how parents care for their children's health in poverty.

Over the last fifty years there has been a proliferation of people, mainly from the field of psychology, who define themselves as childcare 'experts'. There is no shortage of advice or theories for parents or those who work with parents. In much of the literature there is a marked tendency to view children's health and attainment as the outcome of factors within the family. Cultural ideas and practices within the home, childcare ideologies and parental characteristics are seen as crucial variables. Many studies of the 1960s and 1970s have favoured explanations of differences in childcare and child health in terms of social class or cultural practices. The childcare practices of manual social classes and minority ethnic families are often seen as being less health enhancing and less in line with professional advice than the practices of other groups. The lower health status and poorer social and educational attainment of children in poverty is explained in terms of the inappropriate attitudes to health and childcare, or the deviant behaviour of parents, who live in deprived and stressful circumstances.[1]

This perspective also informs studies that have sought to explain the continued presence of poverty and deprivation in a society where standards of living have risen. These ideas form the basis of the 'culture of poverty' explanations. Here poverty is seen to be perpetuated when children internalize values acquired from the family. This theory is closely linked to the 'cycle of deprivation' theory which rests on the assumption that parents bring to the care of their children sets of values and behaviour from their own upbringing. A deficiency of skills in parenthood and undesirable attitudes lead to family problems which tend to recur in future generations. Both the culture of poverty theory and the theory of transmitted deprivation hold that processes within the family, even if maintained by external forces, are responsible for the perpetuation of poverty and deprivation.[2]

The idea that childcare practices are the outcome of factors within the family is also deeply ingrained in the views of many professionals.[3] Much health and welfare work with families focuses on persuading parents to take responsibility for their children's health and welfare and giving them the skills and knowledge to do so. The basis of this work rests on the implicit assumption that parents do not necessarily know how to be good parents and need to be taught appropriate parenting skills. The consequence of these assumptions is that much health and welfare work with parents is problem orientated and based on interventions that seek to identify deficits in the childcare skills and attitudes of parents.

The majority of research studies based on these kinds of assumptions have focused on how parents in different social groups differ in their childcare practices. As a result they have been able to record, in many cases, significant differences between families. Mayall makes the point that it is valuable to distinguish between parents' childcare approaches and their childcare practices. Studies that survey childcare practices will inevitably find differences between social groups. Mayall's study of child health care, by focusing on parents' childcare approaches and what they wish to achieve, found that parents appear to be more similar than different in their attitudes to child health care. She suggests that differences in childcare practices are more likely to reflect the environments in which parents carry out their child health care rather than their attitudes or goals. Here childcare studies share similar findings to studies of health behaviour. If individual behaviour itself is the sole object of study, it is common to record substantial differences between groups. This was clear in chapter 3 of this book which documented how poor families have less healthy diets than higher-income groups. When the focus of studies is extended beyond practices to include goals and attitudes, we find more similarities than differences in outlook across social groups. It is necessary to look behind the practices themselves to what parents with different household incomes aim to and prefer to do. This highlights how childcare practices do not necessarily reflect parental attitudes or skill deficits, but how profoundly child health care is affected by a lack of material health resources.

In keeping with the rest of the book, this chapter is concerned with the way income shapes childcare experiences and practices. To examine the key question 'How does poverty influence the childcare practices of parents?' the chapter will examine the following areas:

- *Parents' attitudes and beliefs about health and health care:* how the concepts of health that parents hold and their childcare goals shape their childcare practices.
- *Patterns of childcare work:* examining how childcare is shaped according to who is involved in child health-care work and the content of this work. It will discuss the personal and material costs of caring.
- *Patterns of caring in health and in sickness:* examining how poverty shapes the way parents care for their children when they are well and when they are sick, and how they use doctors and preventive health services.

PARENTS' ATTITUDES TO HEALTH AND CHILD HEALTH CARE

A common assumption underlying much paid health and welfare work is that parents need to change their attitudes to child health and increase their knowledge about their children's health needs. Mayall and Foster's survey of parents' and health visitors' perspectives on child health-care work documented that many health visitors thought that mothers commonly had poor characteristics for mothering. Mothers tend to be over-anxious, uncaring, lacking confidence, easily led, often immature and lacking fore-thought and forward-planning abilities.[4] Studies suggest that other groups of welfare workers hold similar negative attitudes about parents. Attitudes tend to be most negative towards parents in poverty. Jordan[5] has suggested that, in the case of social work, parents in poverty may have to express their material needs as personal and emotional childcare problems to get help. This section will address whether these assumption about parents, particularly parents in low-income groups, are generally correct.

When all parents carry out their childcare work, they bring to it attitudes, beliefs and knowledge from numerous sources: past and present experiences, friends, relatives, professionals, television, radio, books, magazines, health-education campaign materials and dominant social and political values. The attitudes, beliefs and knowledge that parents hold inform their childcare work in several ways. This section will discuss specifically how parents' childcare work is informed, first, by the concepts of health and illness they hold and, second, by what they wish to achieve in this work. Two more factors, the division of childcare labour and the content of childcare work, will be discussed in the next section.

CONCEPTS OF HEALTH

To establish whether people hold a responsible attitude to health, we need to establish what they mean by the term 'health' in the first place. Concepts of health and illness have been a popular area of study over the last two decades as researchers have recognized the relationship between views about health and the health actions that people carry out or fail to carry out. Studies of adult lay concepts of health have indicated that health can be defined in three main ways: in a negative way, as the absence of illness; functionally, as the ability to cope; positively as a positive state of fitness and well-being.[6]

Studies have found that concepts of health differ between social groups: between people in manual and non-manual occupations, between people with different levels of education and between people of different cultures. Studies have found that people in manual occupations and those who are in less educated groups tend to define health narrowly. These studies suggest that manual classes see health as a more negative or functional concept than non-manual classes and more educated groups. Manual and less educated groups are likely to see health as the absence of disease or ability to cope with everyday life. People in non-manual occupations and groups with higher levels of education tend to see health as a broader and more positive concept.[7,8] For these groups, health is likely to be about more than the absence of disease, and about a sense of well-being. Other studies have indicated that, if different interview techniques are used, differences between social classes are less clear cut. When studies have used interview schedules that have allowed concepts of health to be explored in more depth and have given people more time to become familiar with the interviewer, people in manual occupations have expressed ideas about health that are just as broad and complex as other groups.

Studies show that everyday living experiences shape ideas about health and illness. People select concepts that help them to understand and cope with their own health experiences and the health experiences of others.[9] This approach helps us to understand why people with fewer material health resources and lower health status may hold concepts of health that relate to the absence of disease, or to health as a functional state concerned with 'coping' or 'getting through the day'. These health concepts reflect the life experiences of low-income groups which for many people are about surviving and being able to carry on with the necessities of everyday life.

Culture and ethnicity shape people's concepts of health. Our ideas about health and illness are socially produced. Our cultural and ethnic background influence the health concepts of us all. An examination of culture and ethnicity helps to explain why some groups differ from others in the concepts of health that they hold, and why there may be variance within groups of similar socio-economic positions. Mares *et al.*[10] make the point that many health workers can easily fall into the trap of thinking that concepts of health which are not based on Western, medical science are illogical and invalid. In a multi-ethnic society such as Britain, it is important that health and welfare workers seek to understand the logic and belief systems that people hold. Currer's study of Pathan women in Britain[11] is a good example of how health concepts may differ according to culture. This study highlights how health and illness concepts held by Pathan women have to be understood in terms of Pathan culture and the structural position they occupy in a British society. Currer found that Pathan women viewed health and illness, happiness and unhappiness as part of the same natural order. Being healthy was not an aim or ideal for these women, as it was seen as one's fate. They felt little responsibility for health or illness. Their responsibility, as women in Pathan society, was not to prevent illness, but to behave correctly in the face of illness.

Studies of lay concepts of health have concentrated on how adults view their own health. Mayall's study of white parents' views about child health and child health care examined the concepts of health that mothers held for their children. The parents in Mayall's study described good health for their children as a positive state: it was more than the absence of disease. Health was about reaching their full potential, gaining strength, learning, being talkative, active and investigative. Healthy children were happy children who ate and slept well. A further survey of parents' concepts of health was carried out by Combes and Braun.[12] This study, of predominantly Asian parents and children's understanding of health and illness, also illustrated that parents used complex notions of health and illness. These concepts of health and illness were related to the everyday circumstances of their lives. Like the parents in Mayall's study, the parents in Combes and Braun's study saw a clear connection between children's happiness and their health. Whereas mothers in poor social groups may have more negative ideas about what constitutes health for themselves, their social circumstances may not confine what they view as good health for their children. It may be incorrect to assume that parents' attitudes to child health and childcare can be surmised from attitudes to their own health.

One of the reasons given by health and welfare workers for their pre-occupation with parents' health concepts is the concern that negative health orientations may be picked up by children. This concern, as we saw at the start of this chapter, has also been one shared by 'culture of poverty' theorists and thus is an important issue to consider.

The extent to which health orientations are passed on in families is a question that has aroused the interest of researchers. Whilst some studies have recorded similarities within families, other studies have found otherwise. For example, Blaxter and Paterson studied mothers and daughters in manual occupations in Scotland.[13] They found that there was little direct evidence of the transmission of ideas between mother and daughter and almost no evidence of direct influence on behaviour. Changes in public attitudes to health over time may be more important than transmission of ideas from one generation to another. Campbell[14] has suggested that, where similarities can be found, they can be explained in terms of the fact that, as children grow older, influences outside the family such as school and friends become more important. The fact that parents and children share the same social-class experiences means that they will inevitably share some similar ideas about health and illness.

CHILDCARE GOALS

Research studies question the assumption, held by some health and welfare workers, researchers and politicians, that many parents, particularly those in low-income groups, do not place enough emphasis on health in their childcare work. A growing body of research suggests that parents, regardless of their income group, aim for the same goals in their childcare; they place high emphasis on health in their childcare work and have high standards of health for their children. Parents' childcare goals are likely to be closely linked to the concepts of health they hold for their children. There is strong evidence to suggest that, regardless of social class, all parents, Black or white, all want what is best for their children.[15,16,17] Both Graham and Mayall have documented how parents share similar goals, regardless of their income group or social class. Mothers see all their unpaid activities as work that actively promotes and maintains their children's well-being. Research studies indicate that parents classify all the work they carry out in the home as health work. Parental activities and concerns that are often assumed to be directed to other ends, such as cleaning or washing, are often perceived by mothers as crucial to the promotion of good health in their children. However, many studies of family health care and childcare activities have tended to define tasks narrowly, separating out discrete areas of activity to survey (for example, shopping and food preparation, or housework). By separating out child and family health-care tasks, we end up with a fragmented and incomplete picture. Graham[18] suggests that we need to include in our discussions activities which are often excluded as health-care activities, or taken for granted, such as shopping, cleaning or taking a child to visit friends. Through these activities, parents are providing the physical, emotional and social environment in which their children can grow and develop. Many childcare tasks are carried out simultaneously with other tasks, for example, a shopping trip to buy essential food supplies also gives the child an outing. Mayall's surveys (1986,[19] 1990[20]) of childcare activities found that mothers perceive activities that one might assume were towards other ends as crucial for children's health. They view childcare and child development as taking place within the everyday organization of family life. Health and welfare workers, on the other hand, may hold a different view. Mayall and Foster's study (1990)[21] showed that health visitors appeared to regard child health-care activities as being more purposeful activities that demanded the specific input of adults. This perspective may explain why many contacts between professionals and parents tend to concentrate on a small proportion of childcare activities – those tasks which are directly related to health. Other activities remain invisible to the professional. It is only when professionals are concerned that parents are not providing a suitable environment for their children that they pay attention to servicing activities, such as shopping and cleaning. The way household and childcare tasks and demands are related and need to be reconciled is rarely given attention. The conflicts and compromises involved in this reconciliation will be discussed later in this chapter.

Mayall's study found that all mothers had high standards of health for their children. Nor did they differ in what they thought promoted good health. All mothers emphasized that it was their own care of the child that affected their child's health status. But whilst accepting a personal responsibility for their children's health, mothers described how material constraints affected their ability to carry out this care. Some of these material constraints will be discussed later in this chapter and have been referred to in previous chapters of this book. Combes and Braun's study[22] also draws attention to the way that parents perceive a broad range of factors, such as bullying, rubbish in the locality and pollution, as impacting on children's health. These studies highlight that, when we talk about caring for children, we need to include the broad issues that parents themselves identify as affecting the health of their children.

Whilst mothers have positive goals in their child health-care work, they may have different long- and short-term goals than professionals.[23] Where mothers may give some priority to short-term as well as long-term childcare goals, professionals may be more likely to operate with long-term goals. The mothers in Mayall and Foster's study, who were from a number of ethnic backgrounds, identified two short-term goals as of paramount importance. First, their children's present happiness and the happiness of others in the family were perceived as important. Second, for mothers it was important that their children appeared to be doing well now in comparison to other children. Health visitors were more interested in long-term childcare goals for children. Childcare was good if parents carried out activities that would help the child to do well at school or lead to good health in later life. Both mothers and health visitors considered it important that children reached professionally identified developmental targets. Mothers' concern for their children's present happiness, as well as their future happiness, may explain why some mothers reject or compromise some aspects of professional childcare advice. (The need for mothers to compromise the needs of children will be discussed later in this chapter.)

PATTERNS OF CHILDCARE WORK

To understand how poverty affects child health care, it is necessary to examine the everyday experience of parenting and childcare. For some readers this may appear to be an irrelevant area of investigation. Some people who work with families and/or have children of their own may feel that they already know what this experience involves. There are several reasons why it is valuable to spend a little time discussing this. First, the conditions under which parents care vary according to a number of factors, but primarily according to income and access to material resources. The majority of health and welfare workers will not personally have experienced the conditions under which many low-income families care for their children. Second, we all make assumptions about family life, including the experience of parenting and how parents care for their children. It is important to check that these assumptions fit in with what parents actually experience when they care for their children in and out of poverty. This is particularly important in relation to families from Black and minority ethnic groups. This section will attempt to address the experience of parenting and childcare by first examining who cares for children's health at home, and second, by examining which activities are involved.

It is important to note that many of the studies that inform this section are studies of the experiences of white parents who were born in the UK. We have very little information about how parents from minority ethnic groups experience parenthood. The need to find out more about the factors that shape the childcare practices of families from minority ethnic groups is a key issue for research and practice to address. It is of paramount importance to investigate how living in a white, ethnocentric and often racist society shapes the parenting experiences of Black and minority ethnic parents. The accounts of parents' experiences that we do have suggest that poor Black and minority ethnic parents share many of the social and economic circumstances of poor white parents, plus the additional problems of living in a society that is often unfriendly and hostile to them.

WHO DOES THE CARING?

Several studies have examined the distribution and organization of child health-care work. These studies highlight that child health-care work is firmly divided along gender lines, and differs according to family structure.

Mothers still carry out the vast majority of child health-care work in Britain today. Surveys of child care have tended to identify who does the work rather than to what extent the division of childcare labour has changed over the years. Whilst there is a general consensus that fathers in two-parent families are a little more involved in child health-care activities now than twenty years ago, it is difficult to quantify by how much. The British Social Attitudes Survey which began in 1983 has recorded that there has been very little change in recent years (1983–7) in the amount of housework that fathers do, or their degree of involvement in the two childcare activities measured by the survey.[24] Any increase in male participation in childcare has not matched women's increasing participation in the labour market. There has been a dramatic increase in the number of women who are economically active outside the home:

43 per cent of women aged 15–59 (26 per cent of married women) were in paid employment outside the home in 1951. This has increased to 66 per cent of women aged 16–59 (61 per cent of married women) in 1986.[25]

A large number of families no longer fit the stereotyped image of a nuclear family, with a bread-winning father and a stay-at-home, home-making mother. An increasing number of women now have dual roles: they combine paid work with unpaid caring. For many women, their work outside the home does not significantly decrease the amount of caring work they do in the family. Moreover, the growing number of lone-mother families means that an increasing number of women care for their children's health with no, or only occasional, input from children's fathers. The higher rate of lone motherhood among Afro-Caribbean women than among white, British women means that Afro-Caribbean mothers are particularly likely to be doing this caring alone.

Mothers spend substantially higher proportions of their time than men carrying out child health-care activities, regardless of whether they are in paid employment or not.

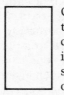

Piachaud's study (1986) of the time costs of childcare indicated that mothers' input accounted for 89 per cent of the total household time spent on childcare activities.[26]

Although Black and white women bear the brunt of child health care in the majority of families, they do not necessarily care unaided. In two-parent families fathers share or assist with child health care activities to varying degrees:

Graham (1986) identified that in-two parent households, 90 per cent of partners helped in some way with child care.[27]

Charles and Kerr's study (1985) of family eating habits and attitudes towards nutrition, involving parents with pre-school children, identified that only 11 per cent of fathers were not involved in childcare activities in two-parent households. Only 11 per cent shared childcare responsibilities and activities equally, and another 12 per cent shared the care when they were not at work.[28]

Mayall (1986) identified that 22 per cent of fathers in households with a white, British-born mother and a first-born child under 36 months shared equally in child health-care activities when they were at home.[29]

Bell, McKee and Priestley's study of fathers, childbirth and work showed that the majority of fathers voiced the view that they wished to participate and share in childcare activities. However, their views about the boundaries of participation and sharing were elastic and shifted widely between fathers.[30] This study indicated that, although mothers carry out the bulk of childcare activities, fathers' participation increases around the time of childbirth. Other studies have identified that fathers in two-parent families are likely to increase their involvement when extra help is needed, for example, if there are many young children in the family, or if mothers are so ill that they cannot carry on.[31]

Other family members and friends also help mothers with children's health care. Other relatives who live in the same household may also contribute to the care of children. Where families live as extended households, there is likely to be more sharing of care between parents and other adults in the household. Some studies have also highlighted how older children may contribute to the care of younger children, often helping out with activities such as playing and baby-sitting. This appears to be particularly the case in large families, where some parenting tasks are delegated to older siblings.[32] People outside the household are also important sources of help for parents. Relatives appear to offer the most practical help: with baby-sitting, child minding and help when children are ill.[33] Studies indicate that a mother's own family, particularly her own parents, tend to have the highest input into the care of children.[34] There is some indication that the lack of help from fathers in lone-mother families is compensated for, to some extent, by higher levels of help from other family members and friends. However, this help is unlikely to cover the areas where fathers in two-parent families are most likely to help: with shopping, putting the child to bed and housework.[35]

Friends also support parents in their childcare activities. Friends do not appear to be substitute carers, as they are usually mothers themselves, but offer short-term assistance when needed. Parents appear to value the social support and advice that friends offer. The amount of help that parents receive from others appears to vary between studies. It is useful to make a distinction between practical forms of help and help in the form of advice and support. Those studies that indicate that parents receive very little help are usually referring to practical help, for example, Piachaud[36] found that 78 per cent of mothers did not have anyone, apart from their partner, to help with the care of children. Other studies have illustrated how parents receive significant amounts of help and support from families and friends.[37,38] One of the most valuable forms of support that other people offer is advice and emotional support. The companionship of friends is particularly valued.

WHAT DOES CARING FOR CHILDREN INVOLVE?

Caring for children is a physical and emotional task. In their role as carers, parents experience a wide variety of emotions. The vast majority of parents, regardless of their social circumstances, stress that loving and interacting with their child are among the most rewarding aspects of their lives. With parenthood comes a new identity and a new sense of responsibility:

You don't realize the responsibility. I think you just think you're going to have this baby and everything's going to stay the same and it doesn't. Everything changes. Even you, your feelings about yourself and you think, 'Well I'm not a girl any more, I'm a mother.' You think this little baby is dependent on you like I was on my mum.

(Mother talking about her feelings after the birth of her first child)[39]

To examine what childcare involves, it is necessary to examine what activities need to be performed. Piachaud offers a framework for analysing the time spent caring for children.[40] It illustrates the breadth of child health activities:

 Basic tasks: activities involving the child (such as bathing, feeding, changing, toileting); servicing activities (including shopping, cleaning, doing the laundry).

 Educational and entertaining tasks.

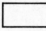 Indirect supervisory and on-call activities.

The range of activities involved in childcare denotes the enormity of the task. Several studies have attempted to calculate the amount of time involved in child health-care activities. These studies indicate that keeping children healthy is a full-time job – twenty-four hours a day, seven days a week:

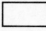 Piachaud calculated that basic childcare tasks alone in families with a pre-school child (see above for Piachaud's framework) take on average, seven hours a day, fifty hours a week.[41]

 Graham's survey identified that mothers spent up to 70 per cent of a fifteen-hour day caring for children.[42]

Graham's survey of the organization of health resources and responsibilities in white families with pre-school children informs us that we also need to extend Piachaud's framework to include activities that parents do for themselves. We need to include activities that parents perform in order to maintain themselves in their caring role, for example, sitting down and having a cup of coffee, or maintaining contact with friends. Graham found that in families with pre-school children:[43]

80 per cent of main activities in the carer's day were directly linked to family health.

A large proportion of the remaining 20 per cent of activities was also related to family health, and included activities that helped to maintain the health of parents.

The amount of time spent on childcare is likely to differ according to the age of the child, the number of children in the household, and whether a mother is living with a partner or not. Parents with a very young child are likely to find themselves having more time-consuming childcare activities than parents with older children. As the number of children in the household increases, so will the number of times parents need to attend to their children. As children grow older, the time spent on carrying out activities for children, such as dressing, washing and toileting, decreases as children learn to carry out these activities for themselves. However, servicing and supervisory responsibilities are likely to continue much longer – for many parents until children leave the family home. The most time-consuming activity for many mothers with young children is feeding, including food preparation, supervising mealtimes and washing-up afterwards. For parents of children with disabilities, the amount of time spent on childcare activities is likely to be increased and the duration when the child is dependent on his or her parents is usually prolonged. In cases of severe disablement, parents may continue to carry out direct health-care tasks, supervisory tasks and servicing activities for the rest of the child's or their own active life.

Studies of the experience of caring for children indicate the nature of everyday caring activities. *First, caring for children's health is heavy, and tiring work.* In Piachaud's study of the time costs of caring in families with a pre-school child:

83 per cent of mothers thought their total childcare workload was more than or equal to a full-time job, without a child.

45 per cent of mothers found the job very tiring, 45 per cent found it tiring, only 9 per cent did not find it tiring.

Unlike paid work, unpaid caring has no official breaks, or officially recognized workloads. As well as the working day being far longer than any full-time paid job, mothers who are caring for children at home have very few breaks away from their pre-school children. Young children frequently go everywhere with their mothers. Where mothers go, children go. The following studies indicate how little time mothers can call their own:

Graham found that the majority of mothers of pre-school children had only 2–4 hours a day to relax, without their children. 12 per cent had less.[44]

Piachaud found that 64 per cent of women had no break of an hour or more a week when they were free from children or paid employment. Only 5 per cent of mothers had one three-hour break per week.

For lone parents, the opportunities to take breaks or opt out of supervisory activities are often limited. At particular times of the day – early morning and early evening – childcare activities appear to be particularly concentrated. These are noted to be crisis times, when the pressures of childcare build up, and nerves are fraught. In two-parent families, these are times when fathers are often present to help out. Lone parents are unlikely to have this help.

Second, caring for children's health is a highly routinized, but constantly changing activity. Approximately 80 per cent of main family health-care activities in both one and two-parent families are likely to be performed each day.[45] A carer's routine is dictated by the needs of the family and the outside world. While some needs and demands must be met, no matter what (children need to be fed regardless of what demands are being made on carers or whatever crisis occurs), others can be put off. The way children's needs and demands are reconciled with the needs and demands of others, and those of everyday life, will be discussed in the section that follows.

CARING IN SICKNESS AND IN HEALTH

On close examination it is clear that all the work that parents do is childcare work. This involves both unpaid activities that directly involve the child, and all other work that parents do in the home. For many parents, particularly working mothers in low-income households, paid work outside the home directly provides the health resources that children need. By its very nature, childcare work is actively concerned with health promotion and disease prevention. As a consequence, when this work fails to prevent illness, childcare work is also about caring in sickness. In real-life situations, activities and roles are not discrete or independent factors. They interlink and are at times in conflict.

The next four sub-sections will examine how parents care for their children in sickness, and how they promote good health, illustrating how their activities and goals are constrained by two issues: lack of choice and the need to make compromises in their childcare work.

CARING FOR CHILDREN IN HEALTH

Parents feel that they are promoting their children's health in everything they do. Health promotion is an integral part of their childcare work. Whilst the majority of parents appear to have the same high standards of health for their children and share childcare goals, their opportunities to reach these standards and goals are affected by the social and economic conditions in which they live.

Control is a major issue in the lives of low-income families. The majority of low-income families are unable to choose where they live, or how they live. Lack of money and other material resources shape both the routines and choices that parents make for their own health and their children's health. Low income and poor housing conditions are two factors that hinder parents' health promotion and disease-prevention activities.

When children are born, the resource needs of families increase, and household costs go up. Yet household income rarely increases in line with needs. Indeed in the majority of families, household income decreases when women stop work to have children. Although families in receipt of social-security benefits receive additional amounts for each child, payments are small and have been shown to be insufficient to meet the health needs of children.[46] Moreover, living conditions that may have been acceptable before the birth of a child may no longer be acceptable once a child is present.

Low income makes it difficult to exercise control and choice over child-care in a number of areas. The difficulties that parents experience in exercising control and choice in areas of healthy eating, keeping warm and home safety, were discussed in previous chapters. The following extract gives some insight into the difficulties that mothers on low income face in their health-promotion work:

> Nine-month-old George had just begun crawling. The lounge is so cramped that he cannot move more than a metre in a straight line without trouble. While Mum is making the tea, he bangs his head on the steel frame of the coffee-table and howls. There is near panic as he touches the white powder on the air ducts: it is insecticide, put there to kill pharaoh ants and cockroaches. Meanwhile Peter, only a year older, falls over a tricycle on to his face and later totters out of the kitchen with a carving knife in his hand.[47]

Whilst parents with low incomes lack choice and control in child health care relative to other families, they are not passive in the face of difficulty. Whilst poverty reduces the amount of power and choice that parents have, they appear to go to great lengths to take control over those parts of their lives which they can control. One of the ways parents do this is by making compromises. Whilst compromise is a common theme in the lives of all families, low-income families experience the greatest and most extensive forms of compromise.

Caring for children's health in poverty involves compromising the needs of parents for the sake of children. In poverty, the sacrifices that parents make for the sake of their children are striking, and have been a recurring theme throughout this book. The following quotations illustrate some common areas of compromise for parents:

> And I think, well these kids are not going to suffer. I'd sooner they had a meal than I had a meal sort of thing.

> I've had two pairs of jeans since I've got married and that's three years. You just don't sort of kit yourself. I'd sooner myself go in jeans than have these [children] go tatty, 'cause it don't look good. I suppose every family is the same.
>
> (Two unemployed fathers talking)[48]

Caring for children's health may also mean compromising one health activity in favour of another. Faced with a tired and irritable child, a mother may decide to put a child to bed, unwashed and without cleaning the child's teeth because, in her eyes, the child's health need for sleep overrides any immediate need to be clean. Parents may fail to take a child to be immunized because he has a runny nose, which is often viewed by parents as a contra-indication. A breast-feeding mother may decide to change to bottle feeding because, as she cannot measure how much milk her infant is receiving, she worries that he/she may not be getting enough food. For a mother, changing to bottle feeding may be a rational decision to protect the health of her baby, even though it may be against the advice of a health worker.

Caring for children's health involves compromising the needs of one child for the needs of other people. Parents have obligations to other people. These obligations may have to take priority over the needs of a particular child or group of children in a household. A parent may have to leave a sick child in the care of another person in order to meet the demands of an employer. Parents in poverty frequently have to compromise the needs of their children to a far greater extent than parents of children in higher-income groups. For example, a growing number of mothers in low-income families feel they have to leave their children to go out to work in order to ensure that a family has an adequate household income. Their choice to work or stay at home is significantly more constrained than mothers in higher-income families. Moreover, a mother may have little option but to leave her child in day-care provision that is not of the standard she desires.

Compromising children's health needs in poverty may be a matter of having no choice:

> The baby could have had better nourishment before he was born if I'd had enough money to be able to eat properly and now I'm breastfeeding he would get better fed if I was.
>
> (Mother of new baby)[49]

Compromising children's health needs may not be a purposeful choice, but a necessary decision that is taken to maintain peace and harmony in the home. Graham has documented how mothers balance the needs of one child against the needs of others in the family.[50] For example, she may reject child health-care advice from health and welfare workers, because to follow that advice would be to sacrifice the needs of others. The early introduction of solids may pacify a hungry baby who wakes at night and needs frequent feeds. This, in turn, may allow a mother to spend more time meeting the needs of other family members or let others sleep. Furthermore, parents may sacrifice the needs of individual children in order to preserve harmonious relations with people outside the home. Wilson and Herbert[51] found that the collective needs of a neighbourhood may take priority over the needs of individuals in families. In certain types of housing, where proximity of neighbours and lack of play space are evident, the need to maintain good relationships with neighbours may prevent parents from allowing their children to play certain types of games or from playing outdoors. When parents fail to make this latter type of compromise, they are often labelled as irresponsible parents. It is clear that the behaviour of parents in poverty and many of their childcare choices are not free choices but choices that are constrained by parents' sense of responsibility for others, and the material and social circumstances under which they live.

USE OF PREVENTIVE SERVICES

Childcare practices in the home form a significant part of child health-care activities, but not the total sum. Caring for children in health also involves contact with child health services. It is often assumed that parents' attitudes and lack of knowledge act as a barrier towards use of child health services. Research into the utilization of preventive health services has been far less extensive in Britain than in the United States, and studies that do exist have recorded how utilization patterns differ between groups, without necessarily examining why they differ. Studies from the United States indicate that preventive health-care services appear to be least used by lower socio-economic groups, whether utilization is recorded according to income, education or occupation. Although findings from these studies cannot automatically be expected to explain British patterns of utilization of preventive health services, they are important in that they indicate that explanatory models that rest on individual or social factors alone are inadequate. Whether individuals use preventive health services or not seems to depend on interrelated factors. Moreover, these studies suggest that, rather than looking at the characteristics of poor attenders of preventive services, it is more useful to examine factors that act as barriers or enablers to service use.

Child health clinics offer one of the main preventive health services for children. Although child health clinics now tend to describe themselves as a resource for parents, they are predominantly places where mothers go. However, it is perhaps a little more common to see fathers in a child health clinic now than it was ten years ago. Several studies have highlighted that mothers appear to use the clinic if they see it as meeting a need that cannot be met elsewhere. Mothers value child health clinics as an advice resource, and for its role in child health screening and surveillance. They attend to be reassured that their children are progressing well, to gain advice, and to meet other mothers.[52,53] Mothers with very young children, particularly first-time mothers, appear to use clinics the most.[54] Attendances appear to decline rapidly once children reach one year of age. It is suggested that as mothers become more confident in their parenting role, and more knowledgeable about the needs of their children, they no longer feel they need to attend the clinic as frequently. This may also explain why mothers tend to use the clinic more frequently with their first child than they do with subsequent children, and why mothers with older children feel that they no longer need to attend as frequently. Studies have also indicated that mothers with low levels of social support tend to use child health clinics the most. For these mothers, chatting with a health visitor at a clinic may meet a need that is met by families and friends for other mothers. For mothers who have recently moved into a new neighbourhood or into the country from abroad, clinics can be extremely valuable sources of support if they provide services that overcome cultural and language barriers and if the staff are sufficiently welcoming.

Health and welfare workers often assume that those who would most benefit from using child health clinics, that is, groups with high levels of disadvantage, often use them the least. There appears to be some confusion about which social groups underutilize child health clinics. Several studies have indicated that there is little difference in patterns of use by social class,[55,56] whilst others have recorded under use by manual social classes.[57] The Child Health and Education Study[58] found little differences in patterns of attendance by social class but, by using a measure of social disadvantage, the social index, it identified that the children of those who had the highest disadvantage scores attended clinics the least. This study indicated that a low number of clinic attendances among groups with high social disadvantage may to some extent, be compensated for by more home-visits from health visitors.

There is some evidence to suggest that it may be incorrect to assume that those groups with the most needs have the worst attendance rates. Morgan et al.'s study[59] of the use of child health clinics in inner-city areas indicated that comparing the use of clinics by levels of deprivation may be too simplistic. Morgan's study illustrates the usefulness of looking at the characteristics of neighbourhoods in relation to use of child health services. Attendances at child health clinics from parents from the poorest council estates were higher than expected. They had higher attendance rates than parents from mixed metropolitan areas (areas with high numbers of people born overseas) and high status inner-city areas (more prosperous areas). Higher attendance levels among mothers from the poorest council estates may reflect the higher levels of unmet needs. More children from this group were identified as having unsatisfactory findings at the seven-month developmental screening check, and higher numbers of children needed to see the doctor. This study indicated that groups with the greatest need appeared to have the highest attendance rates.

In the absence of any firm evidence on patterns of use of child health clinics, it is useful to examine which barriers may discourage some groups from attending. Studies have predominantly studied barriers which discourage white parents. Whilst poor clinic attendance by Black and minority ethnic families is viewed as a problem and often portrayed as reflecting their failure to act responsibly, research has failed to comment on the barriers that prevent or discourage Black and minority ethnic families from using preventive services.

Many mothers value child health screening and surveillance checks, but there is evidence to suggest that they do not use clinics unless they feel it is necessary to do so. Rather than reflecting a negative attitude to preventive services, this may reflect that mothers feel they are able to assess for themselves whether their children are developing well or not. It has been well documented that parents are sensitive observers of their children and often detect abnormalities in their children and bring them to the attention of professionals.[60] There is evidence that some mothers are confused about the role of child health clinics, and how they differ from family-doctor services. Lack of information about the need for screening checks and the time schedule of the checks have been shown to be a further barrier to use of clinics.[61] Some mothers have also expressed a concern about the way professionals control information at child health clinics. Mothers dislike not being able to see what health visitors and doctors are writing about their children. Other mothers have expressed a concern that checks were not always performed to a high standard and often failed to tell them anything they did not already know about their child.[62] Indeed, the value of frequent screening and surveillance checks, particularly if they are not performed to a high standard, have been questioned by child-care experts. It has been suggested that less frequent, but more thorough screening checks would be more effective in identifying children with unmet health needs.[63]

Although children from socially disadvantaged groups would most benefit from preventive health services, in view of their higher illness rates, it appears that they often live in areas that have the least encouraging facilities. Spencer and Power's study of the characteristics of clinics in Nottingham[64] indicated that clinics in deprived areas were least likely to be able to offer services that met needs because they were likely to be overstretched:

Clinics in deprived areas had more children registered with them than clinics in non-deprived areas.

A large number of children at clinics in deprived areas presented with medical problems.

Other studies have identified further barriers and deterrents to the use of child health services. Some studies have identified that the distance that mothers have to travel to clinic and the times of clinic sessions are a barrier[65] and others have identified that mothers may be put off by the formality of child health clinics. As one of the reasons mothers give for attending child health clinics is a desire to meet other mothers and children, if the organization of sessions does not allow this, then mothers will perceive that clinics no longer meet their needs and modify their attendance. The value of making clinic facilities welcoming and convenient to use has been demonstrated and shown to be a way of increasing clinic attendance among poor attenders.[66]

The need to make services more acceptable to minority ethnic groups is of paramount importance. Mothers from minority ethnic groups experience the barriers to service use that white mothers do, and more. Many mothers from minority ethnic groups experience serious difficulties using child health services that are predominantly run by white workers in such a way that white people are most likely to be able to gain advice. Communication difficulties and language differences are significant barriers to using the service. Trained interpreters are rarely available. A further barrier is that health service staff often fail to understand the information needs or cultural expectations of parents from minority ethnic groups. Watson's study of health-service use by mothers with children under two years, from different ethnic groups, indicated that some parents from minority ethnic groups who were born outside the UK were unfamiliar with the benefits of child-health preventive services because they were unavailable in their country of origin.[67]

Use of immunization services and dental services are two more areas of preventive health care for children. It is not possible to discuss use of these services in any depth in this chapter, but it is worth noting that immunization uptake rates and use of dental services are generally thought to follow similar patterns to uptake of child health-clinic services. Regardless of social group, parents appear to have positive attitudes to dental and immunization services, although socially disadvantaged social groups appear to use services less than other groups. The lessons that can be learnt from studies of utilization and consumer views about child health clinics also apply to immunization and dental-services provision.

CARING FOR CHILDREN IN SICKNESS

The same factors that constrain parents when they care for their well children also shape how they care for their children when they are sick. Caring for sick children has been found to be a commoner event in low-income homes than in higher-income homes. As we saw in chapter 2, poverty and health are interlinked, with children from low-income groups having higher illness rates than children from wealthier homes. Parents in low-income households are more likely, at any one point in time, to be caring for a child who is not well, or who has a disability. Moreover, parents in low-income families are more likely to be unwell themselves.

Caring for sick children involves a variety of costs. There are money costs: money for special foods and drinks, extra bedding, extra heating, telephone charges, and the transport costs of visits to family doctors and hospitals. In many low-income families the money costs of caring for a sick child will stretch family resources to the limit. Low income means that some of the sick child's needs will not be met. For example, a child's need to be able to rest quietly is not always possible in families with several young children, and in cramped housing conditions. Other needs may be met by running up households bills which may prove difficult to pay later (for example, heating bills), by borrowing from family and friends or, more commonly, by compromising the needs of other family members. Mothers commonly sacrifice food and clothing to provide a sick child with the resources to restore his or her health.

On top of the material costs of caring for a sick child, it is necessary to add the time and emotional costs of caring. As we saw earlier, many mothers physically care for their sick child with limited input from others. Nursing a sick child not only extends the length of the childcare work day, it also increases the number and intensity of the activities that have to be performed. In poor living conditions, caring for a sick child is likely to be physically and emotionally arduous for parents. Mayall's study of child health-care work identified that families who had poor material resources and had children who had persistent illness were most likely to have problems caring for sick children.[68]

For parents of children with disabilities, the emotional and material costs of caring for children may be prolonged. Many children with disabilities have constant daily nursing needs but also suffer frequent illnesses that need attention from parents and health-care workers. Disability often stretches household financial resources to the limit. Baldwin's study[69] of the costs of caring for disabled children highlights how caring for disabled children can pose extensive financial problems for families. Yet social-security payments for children with disabilities fail to compensate parents for either the day-to-day costs of caring, the extra costs of caring in times of sickness or for lost income when mothers are unable to take up paid employment.

Parents manage the majority of children's illness without any input from professionals. The decision to seek help depends on a number of factors, including how serious parents perceive the symptoms to be, their perception of their own ability to manage the symptoms, the opportunities they have to discuss the symptoms with others, and the number of illnesses that a child has. When parents no longer feel they can manage the symptoms alone, or feel the symptoms signal something more serious, they seek professional advice and/or help. Studies indicate that parents are most likely to seek help in times of illness during the first few years of the child's life, when illnesses can quickly become life threatening, and with a first-born child. This is the time when parents are least able to put a label on the illness themselves or know the appropriate action to take. During the early years of parenthood, parents begin to build up a picture of what a child looks like when he or she is ill, the meaning of symptoms and what action they should take to avoid deterioration and aid recovery. They build up this knowledge from a number of sources, including their experience with their own child, from their interactions with professionals, from discussing symptoms and illness with family and friends and from books and television. Social support and advice from family and friends has been shown to exert a strong influence on parents' ability to manage illnesses themselves or seek help. For mothers with low levels of social support, the opportunities to discuss illness and gain knowledge from family and friends are limited. Family-doctor consultation rates and child health-clinic attendances have both been shown to be higher amongst this group of mothers.[70] Mothers are also more likely to consult when they have a child that has persistent ill health.

USE OF CURATIVE SERVICES

There has been far less research on the use of curative services for children than for adults, and less research in Britain than in the United States. Moreover, British research is hindered, to some extent, by the fact that it has tended to record utilization rates without always seeking to explain why some groups use some services and not others. Research that has concentrated on utilization rates, or the content, rather than on the context of service use has often failed to explain patterns of service use by disadvantaged families, particularly Black and minority ethnic families.

A review of research studies on utilization of curative services shows a mixed picture of concerns on the part of professionals. On the one hand, there is concern about the failure or delay of some social groups, usually manual social classes, to seek help for their children in times of illness. On the other hand, there appears to be concern about the inappropriate use or overuse of some services by manual social classes. Accident and emergency services have frequently been identified as services that are misused by parents. Roberts' study[71] of professionals' and parents' perceptions of accident and emergency department use illustrates that what may be the most most appropriate source of medical attention at the time for a parent may be labelled as the most inappropriate form of attention by medical and nursing staff. When parents who experience difficulties contacting a family doctor try to be 'good' parents by not taking chances with the health of a child through seeking help at the hospital, they may be labelled as over anxious, time wasting and 'bad' parents.

People who have not grown up in Britain may experience further barriers to the effective use of curative services. They may have experienced different kinds of health-care systems and be used to different types of referral and utilization patterns. Black and ethnic-minority families also have to cope with a health service that fails to provide services that meet their specific health needs. For example, it is estimated that about one in four hundred people of Afro-Caribbean and African origin have sickle cell disease, yet screening and counselling services remain vastly inadequate.[72]

It is difficult to draw any firm conclusions from the studies on utilization of curative services for sick children. The overall pattern seen in adults, whereby consultation rates are higher for those from the working class, is lacking in relation to children.[73] The discrepancy between adult and child consultation rates needs further research, since it does not reflect the increased morbidity suffered by children in low-income groups. Mayall found that family-doctor consultation rates were higher in low-income families who had children with persistent illness[74]. Mothers with persistently ill children from social classes III, IV and V contacted their family doctor more frequently than mothers with persistently ill children from social classes I and II. Mayall concluded that this was likely to reflect the additional worries and constraints that caring for a sick child in poor conditions brings.

It is clear that more research needs to examine what constrains families from seeking help from their doctor when their child is ill and what encourages then to seek such help. In addition to the time and material constraints to seeking help, the quality of the service provided may influence whether parents use their family-doctor services. There is no evidence that parents do not consult family doctors because they are dissatisfied with the nature of the consultation, although other factors such as long waiting times and discriminating treatment do appear to play a part.

There is some evidence that families who are materially and socially disadvantaged are more likely to be living in areas where the family-doctor and other health services are poor. For example, poor families are disproportionately concentrated in inner-city and deprived urban areas. Family-doctor premises in these areas often reflect the social and economic conditions of the areas themselves. Surgeries are less likely to be purpose built or well equipped. Families who live in deprived areas are more likely to experience difficulties contacting their own doctor outside surgery hours. Doctors who work in deprived areas are likely to live outside the area and thus use deputizing services more often. Single-handed practices also need to use deputizing services often. Parental dissatisfaction with family-doctor deputizing services is one reason that parents give for using hospital accident and emergency departments for primary care. In Mayall's study it was notable that mothers who were registered with single- or double-handed family-doctor practices and mothers without a telephone were more likely to use the hospital in times of illness than other mothers.

 Jarman found that the percentage of single-handed family doctors was significantly higher in inner-city health districts (between 15–25 per cent) than the average for England (5 per cent).[75]

CONCLUSION AND IMPLICATIONS FOR PRACTICE

Most general surveys of childcare practices have focused on white families, and therefore there is little data on the childcare practices and experiences of Black and minority ethnic families. However, the limited sources of data we do have suggest that Black and minority ethnic families share the same positive childcare goals as their white counterparts. Moreover, their social and economic position means that they share many of the same experiences of parenting as white, low-income families. Poverty, poor housing and poor access to good childcare facilities outside the home means that for Black and white families alike, caring for children's health effectively is an extremely difficult task. The need to examine the barriers that Black and ethnic minority parents experience over and above those of white parents is an issue of paramount importance for both research and practice, but one that has received little attention so far.

This chapter has discussed how parents care for their children's health in poverty. Working with families with young children inevitably involves making value judgements about families. An ideology in which the child-care practices of parents are seen to stem from poor knowledge, failure to hold acceptable attitudes or parental failure to acknowledge childcare responsibilities has set the boundaries for much health and welfare work. The logical conclusion of this perspective is that the responsibility of workers is to improve the attitudes and skills of parents. However, as this chapter has shown, an examination of the research evidence fails to support the assumption that some groups of parents, particularly poor parents, have less health-enhancing and less virtuous attitudes to childcare than others. Parents, regardless of their income, ethnic/cultural background or social class, appear to start off holding very positive attitudes to childcare and child health. The sense of responsibility they feel is reflected in their belief that all their work is child health work. Parents hold very positive and broad concepts of health for their children. Childcare practices cannot be ex-plained only in terms of factors within the family. For whilst parental characteristics and childcare ideologies clearly affect practices, poverty and poor access to material resources appear to have a powerful influence on the childcare practices of parents.

Whilst parents appear to hold similar child-health and childcare goals, their ability to reach these goals is shaped by several factors. Gender and family structure appear to shape the contours of childcare. Unfortunately we know very little about how ethnicity and culture affect the distribution of child health-care work or the nature of the activities themselves, but in most families in Britain women still shoulder many of the time, material and personal costs of childcare. The costs appear to be the greatest for mothers in families with low incomes, particularly lone mothers, and mothers with children with disabilities. The sacrifices that women make in their role as the main care givers to children affects their physical and mental health and affects their long-term employment status. For many women the financial costs of maternity leave, periods away from paid work and periods of part-time work are great.

The nature of parenting itself, complicated by the reality of living in poverty, means that childcare practices stem from a complex decision-making process. When we consider them within the context of the everyday experiences of families, these decisions are neither irrational, nor the product of ignorance. The evidence suggests that, if health and welfare workers wish to work more effectively with families, they must question some of the assumptions they make about families, the nature of family life and the factors that shape childcare practices. First, this evidence highlights that we need to listen to what parents say they want to achieve for their children and what they say prevents them from meeting these goals. We need to respect the wishes of parents, and acknowledge that parents act in the best interests of their child and within the material constraints of their lives. Childcare advice and support to parents need to be realistic and achievable for parents in poverty. As we saw in chapter 3, the content of much healthy-eating advice and literature does not reflect the fact that a growing proportion of families have low incomes. Health and welfare work also needs to focus on parents' own goals and agendas rather than those of agencies. The evidence in this chapter suggests that parents have agendas and goals that are positive and reflect their worries and concerns.

Second, health and welfare workers need to consider the barriers within their own services that work against parents using both the curative and preventive child-health services. Health and welfare services need to offer a flexible and responsive service that meets the needs of parents in the locality. The location, times, quality and content of the service are factors that have the most profound effects on the use of services. These are factors that can be addressed by workers and their managers, without necessarily needing substantial resources. The need to address the language and cultural barriers that prevent minority ethnic groups from using the services need to be seriously considered and addressed. Evidence from projects that have attempted to make child health services more attractive and easy to use have shown how valuable such attempts can be.

Third, health and welfare workers need to consider the nature of their relationship with their clients. Health and welfare workers often talk of giving individuals back responsibility for their health and control over it. Yet, the evidence in this chapter suggests that the responsibility for child health does lie with parents. Parents recognize this responsibility and exercise it on a daily basis. Neither do professionals have control over the childcare work of parents, except perhaps in extreme cases of child-protection work. To a large extent, parents decide what they will do for their children. Professionals only make a small input to the totality of childcare work. Whilst professionals may not have the power over their clients that they think they have, they are able to exercise some control over the amount of information that parents can have access to. Throughout many accounts of childcare, parents have expressed a concern that professionals do not share information with them. The recognition that parents are the main primary health-care givers implies that parents have the right to information about their own and their children's health. It is pertinent to note that only in a few areas of the country do parents have access to and hold their own child's health records. Acknowledging that the majority of low-income parents do a good job in the face of great adversity opens up the way for workers and parents to work together in partnership.

Last, the evidence in this chapter illustrates that many parents need higher incomes and healthier living environments to carry out their child-care work to the standard they desire. Workers may feel that they have no role to play in this. But people who work with families have the knowledge, the professional duty and the power-base to inform government and policy-makers about the implications of present policies for childcare and child health. The need for family policies that recognize the resource needs of parents has been well documented by anti-poverty groups.[76] Anti-poverty research has stressed the need for realistic household incomes through increases in child benefit, income support and family credit, housing policies that reflect the housing needs of parents and the development of employment policies and day-care provision that recognize the childcare commitments of parents.

REFERENCES

1 Mayall, B. (1986). *Keeping Children Healthy.* London, Allen & Unwin.
2 Brown, M. and Madge, N. (1982). *Despite The Welfare State.* London, Heinemann.
3 Mayall, B. and Foster, M.-C. (1990). *Child Health Care: Living With Children, Working For Children.* Oxford, Heinemann Nursing.
4 Mayall, B. and Foster, M.-C. (1990). *ibid.*
5 Jordan, B. (1988). 'Poverty, social work and the state', in Becker, S. and MacPherson, S. (eds). *Public Issues, Private Pain.* London, Insight.
6 Blaxter, M. (1990). *Health and Lifestyles.* London, Routledge.
7 Pill, R. and Stott, N. (1982). 'Concepts of illness causation and responsibility: some preliminary data from a sample of working class mothers' *Social Science and Medicine,* 16: 43–52.
8 d'Houtard, A. and Field, M. (1984). 'The image of health: variations in perceptions of social class in a French population' *Sociology of Health and Illness,* 6: 30–60.
9 Stacey, M. (1986). 'Concepts of health and illness and the division of labour in health care', in Currer, C., Stacey, M. (eds) *Concepts of Health, Illness and Disease.* Leamington Spa, Berg Publishers.
10 Mares, P., Henley, A. and Baxter, C. (1985). *Health Care in Multiracial Britain.* Cambridge, Health Education Council/National Extension College.
11 Currer, C. (1986). 'Concepts of mental well- and ill-being: the case of Pathan mothers in Britain', in Currer, C., Stacey, M. (eds) *Concepts of Health, Illness and Disease.* Leamington Spa, Berg Publishers.
12 Combes, G. and Braun, D. (1989). *Everything Gives You Heart Attacks These Days.* A Report to the Health Education Authority, Community Education Development Centre, Coventry.

13 Blaxter, M. and Paterson, E. (1983). 'The health behaviour of mothers and daughters', in Madge, N. (ed.) *Families at Risk*. London, Heinemann.

14 Campbell, J. (1975). 'Illness is a point of view: the development of children's concepts of illness' *Child Development*, 46: 92–100.

15 Watson, E. (1984). 'Health of infants and use of health services by mothers of different ethnic groups in East London' *Community Medicine*, 6: 127–35.

16 Mayall, B. and Foster, M.-C. (1990). op. cit.

17 Mayall, B. (1986). op. cit.

18 Graham, H. (1986). *Caring For The Family*. London, Health Education Council.

19 Mayall, B. (1986). op. cit.

20 Mayall, B. and Foster, M.-C. (1990). op. cit.

21 Mayall, B. and Foster, M.-C. (1990). op. cit.

22 Combes, G. and Braun, D. (1989). op. cit.

23 Mayall, B. and Foster, M.-C. (1990). op. cit.

24 Jowell, R., Witherspoon, S. and Brook, L. (eds) (1988). *British Social Attitudes*, Fifth Report, 1988/1989. Aldershot, Gower.

25 Jowell, R. *et al.* (1988). *ibid.*

26 Piachaud, D. (1986). *Round About 50 Hours a Week: The Time Costs of Childcare*. London, Child Poverty Action Group.

27 Graham, H. (1986). op. cit.

28 Charles, N. and Kerr, M. (1985). *Attitudes Towards The Feeding And Nutrition Of Young Children*, Research Report no. 4. London, Health Education Council.

29 Mayall, B. (1986). op. cit.

30 Bell, C., McKee, L. and Priestley, K. (1983). *Fathers, Childbirth and Work*. Manchester, Equal Opportunities Commission.

31 Osborn, A., Butler, N. and Morris, A. (1984). *The Social Life of Britain's Five-Year Olds: A Report of the Child Health and Education Survey*. London, Routledge & Kegan Paul.

32 Wilson, H. and Herbert, G. W. (1978). *Parents and Children in the Inner City*. London, Routledge & Kegan Paul.

33 Willmot, P. (1987). *Friendship Networks and Social Support*. London, Policy Studies Institute.

34 Bell, C., *et al.* (1983). op. cit.

35 Osborn, A. *et al.* (1984). op. cit.

36 Piachaud, D. (1986). op. cit.

37 Willmot, P. (1987). op. cit.

38 Mayall, B. (1986). op. cit.

39 Curtice, L. (1989). *The First Year of Life*. London, Maternity Alliance.

40 Piachaud, D. (1986). op. cit.

41 Piachaud, D. (1986). op. cit.

42 Graham, H. (1986). op. cit.

43 Graham, H. (1986). op. cit.

44 Graham, H. (1986). op. cit.

45 Graham, H. (1986). op. cit.

46 Oppenheim, C. (1990). *The Costs of a Child*. London, Child Poverty Action Group.

47 Harrison, P. (1985). *Inside the Inner City*. Harmondsworth, Penguin.

48 McKee, L. (1985). '"We just sort of struggle on" – having a family in the face of unemployment', *Born Unequal*. London, Maternity Alliance.

49 Salfield, A. and Durward, L. (1985). 'Coping, but only just – families' experiences of pregnancy and childbirth on the dole', *Born Unequal*. London, Maternity Alliance.

50 Graham, H. (1984). *Women, Health and the Family*. Brighton, Wheatsheaf.

51 Wilson, H. and Herbert, G. W. (1978). op. cit.

52 Cubbon, J. (1987). 'Consumer attitudes to child health clinics' *Health Visitor*, vol. 60, 6: 185–6.

53 Sefi, S. and MacFarlane, A. (1985). 'Child health clinics: why mothers attend' *Health Visitor*, vol. 58, 5: 129–30.

54 Morgan, W., Reynolds, A. and Morris, R. *et al.* (1989). 'Who uses child health clinics and why?' *Health Visitor*, vol. 62, 8: 244–7.

55 Mayall, B. (1986). op. cit.

56 Osborn, A., *et al.* (1984). op. cit.

57 Davie, R., Butler, N. and Goldstein, H. (1972). *From Birth to Seven: A Report of the Child Development Study*. London, Longman.

58 Osborn, A., *et al.* (1984). op. cit.

59 Morgan, W., *et al.* (1989). op. cit.

60 Spencer, N. J. (1984). 'Parents' recognition of the ill child', in Macfarlane, J. A. (ed.) *Progress in Child Health*, vol. 1. Edinburgh, Churchill Livingstone.

61 Mayall, B. and Foster, M.-C. (1990). op. cit.

62 Mayall, B. and Foster, M.-C. (1990). op. cit.

63 Hall, D. (1989). *Health for All Children*. Oxford, Oxford University Press.

64 Spencer, N. and Power, S. (1978). *Nottingham Child Health Survey*, Occasional Paper 14. Leverhulme Health Education Project, Nottingham University.

65 Betts, G. and Betts, J. (1990). 'Establishing a child health clinic in a deprived area' *Health Visitor*, vol. 63, 4: 2–124.

66 Betts, G. and Betts, J. (1990). *ibid.*

67 Watson, E. (1984). op. cit.

68 Mayall, B. (1986). op. cit.

69 Baldwin, S. (1985). *The Costs of Caring: Families With Disabled Children*. Routledge & Kegan Paul.

70 Mayall, B. (1986). op. cit.

71 Roberts, H. (1990) 'Professionals' and parents' perceptions of accident and emergency use in a children's hospital'. Paper available from Social Paediatric and Obstetric Research Unit, 1 Lilybank Gardens, Glasgow, G12 RZ.

72 Mares, P. *et al.* (1985). op. cit.

73 Blaxter, M. (1981). *The Health of Children*. London, Heinemann Educational.

74 Mayall, B. (1986). op. cit.

75 Jarman, B. (1989). 'General practice', in White, A. (ed.) *Health in the Inner City*. Oxford, Heinemann Medical.

76 Oppenheim, C. (1990). *The Costs of a Child*. London, Child Poverty Action Group.

7 | CONCLUSIONS AND IMPLICATIONS FOR POLICY AND PRACTICE

INTRODUCTION

The book has been concerned with exploring the impact of poverty on the health of families with young children. Family poverty has increased significantly over the last decade, and there is no indication that the 1990s will see a significant decline in the number of families bringing up children on low incomes and in adverse living conditions. This growth in family poverty has underlined the need for health and welfare workers to understand, and respond more effectively to, the needs of families in poverty.

This book has focused on the central question 'Does poverty affect the health of families who experience it, and if so, how?' To address this question, we have had to address a series of other questions along the way. These have included questions about the meaning and causes of poverty for individuals and society. We have attempted to address the question of the distribution of poverty between various social groups in British society – between men and women, between parents and children, between people of different ethnic groups and between different income groups. We have also addressed the question of whether family health is ultimately the outcome of individual health choices and behaviours, or more closely associated with the social and economic conditions in which people live. These questions have, in turn, led to an examination of the assumptions that underlie health and welfare work with families and an assessment of the extent to which these assumptions are valid.

Whilst the book has provided some answers to these questions, it acknowledges that answers are often hard to find. Research and literature on the impact of family poverty on health remain an area for further extensive research. One of the purposes of this book has been not only to answer questions but also, where there are no definitive answers, to stimulate debate. The book has identified the need for more research into the direct effect of income changes on the health of parents and children. We also need to explore why some low-income families are able to cope better than others in similar circumstances. We need to find out more about how particular kinds of social support appear to protect some families from the worst effects of poverty.

It is clear that many studies of poverty, health and family life concentrate on the experiences and health status of white families. This book raises questions about the legitimacy of research and fieldwork approaches that fail to address the needs of Black and minority ethnic families in a multi-ethnic society such as Britain. Whilst some studies have begun to address the social and economic issues that influence how Black and minority ethnic families care for their health, there is still a dearth of material in this area. There are virtually no data on the distribution of resources within Black and minority ethnic families. There is little research either on the crucial question of how experiences of personal and institutional racism affect health. The need to identify the social-support needs of Black and minority ethnic parents and children is particularly important.

This final chapter summarizes the main findings of the book and draws some conclusions. It will do this by:

- Summarizing the evidence on the impact of family poverty on health.
- Identifying the key issues for health and welfare practice and social policy.

FAMILY POVERTY AND HEALTH

THE POVERTY PROBLEM

We began at the start of the book by addressing the question 'What is poverty?' From the evidence it was clear that we need to see poverty as a relative concept. Poverty is not just about what is needed to stay alive, but also about the conditions that allow people to stay healthy and participate in society. Poverty is about being poor relative to other people.

The idea that poverty needs to be viewed as a relative concept has formed the basis of this book. In working with a relative view of poverty, it is clear that poverty is an extensive social and political problem in Britain today, particularly among families with young children. Our discussion of the meaning and extent of poverty in Britain today led us to address the question 'What creates poverty in a relatively prosperous industrial society?' Family poverty appears to be inextricably linked to economic policies and social policies, particularly employment and wage policies and income mainten-ance policies. This book systematically documented how many women, families headed by lone mothers, Black and minority ethnic groups, people with disabilities and people from manual social classes have poor access to income and material resources for health. As a consequence, these groups tend to be disproportionately represented among those in poverty.

Personal accounts of experiences of poverty have been included throughout this book. They provide us with graphic portrayals of how profoundly poverty affects family life and family health. These accounts informed us that, above all, poverty is an experience that permeates every part of family life. Family poverty means living in conditions that are distressing, unhealthy, unsafe and stressful. Poverty is not only about 'doing without' material resources, but also about the lack of opportunities for social relationships, fulfilment and feelings of security. Whilst individuals and families share some common experiences of poverty, the experience of poverty is not the same for all individuals and families. The materials on which we have drawn suggest that men and women, Black and white people, and one- and two-parent families have different experiences of poverty. Racism and sexism, two factors that create poverty and inequality, also influence how poverty is experienced by individuals and families.

POVERTY AND ILL HEALTH

Chapter 1 looked at the evidence that indicated that family poverty is an extensive social problem in Britain. Chapter 2 moved on to examine the question 'What are the links between poverty and health?' The material reviewed in chapter 2 pointed to a strong link between poverty and ill health. Poverty is not only a cause of ill health, but ill health can also bring about poverty. From this, taken together with the information from chapter 1, it was possible to see that people in manual social classes, women and people from Black and minority ethnic groups not only have the lowest incomes, but also the poorest health at all life stages.

Whilst it is clear that the nature of the relationship between poverty and health is an under-developed area of research, the information we have suggests that there is a direct link (although we do not yet know whether it is a causal link) between poverty and poor health. First, the research indicated that social-class differences in health appear to represent differences in income levels between groups. Second, it indicated that widening social-class inequalities in health since the early 1950s appear to be related to trends in relative poverty. As relative poverty levels have increased, so have health inequalities between social groups. This evidence reinforces the view that we need to work with a relative view of poverty. With overall rises in living standards over the century, death rates for the poor have not fallen as fast as death rates for the rich. Being healthy appears to require more than an absolute level of income to stay alive. It requires having a level of income relative to other people which allows families to enjoy similar living standards and participate in similar ways as groups with higher incomes.

The evidence that low-income groups have poorer health than their better-off counterparts is difficult to dispute. However, there remains a great deal of controversy over the reasons for these differences. Hereditary factors and health-selection explanations appeared to offer few insights into why health inequalities exist and have persisted in a relatively prosperous society. This led us to address the major question: 'Do the health effects of poverty stem from the failure of poor families to adopt a healthy lifestyle and choose healthy behaviours, or do they stem from the fact that low-income families lack the financial and material resources for good health?' Chapters 3, 4, 5 and 6 discussed the extent to which low-income families can be held responsible for their high death and illness rates.

HEALTH KNOWLEDGE AND ATTITUDES

Poor knowledge about the content and value of healthy behaviours or undesirable attitudes to health are two reasons commonly cited to account for high rates of ill health and death amongst low-income families. The poor health of Black and minority ethnic families in poverty has frequently been blamed on these factors. This book has questioned the adequacy of such explanations. A growing body of evidence suggests that low levels of health knowledge, undesirable health attitudes and health orientations are not responsible for poor health among families in poverty.

First, low-income families appear to have similar levels of knowledge to other families. Whilst this does not mean that families necessarily possess high levels of health knowledge, it indicates that differences in levels of health knowledge cannot explain the poorer health status of low-income families. Second, there was no evidence to suggest that low-income families necessarily had less desirable health attitudes than other income groups. As a group, low-income families hold positive health concepts and health orientations. This was particularly true in relation to the health of children. All parents, regardless of income or ethnic group, appear to hold very positive attitudes to childcare and child health, and these are reflected in the care they give to them.

BUDGETING AND MONEY MANAGEMENT

A third explanation commonly invoked, and which underlies much health and welfare work, is that families in poverty have poor health because they squander away their income, either through poor budgeting skills or through irresponsible spending patterns. Studies of money management and budgeting strategies in low-income families provide no evidence to support this view. On the contrary, studies of budgeting patterns suggest that, within the limitations of low-income levels, families manage their income and expenditure efficiently. Low-income families allocate a greater proportion of their household expenditure to essential health resources than higher-income families do. The idea that low-income households spend their income recklessly appears to stem, first, from the assumption that poverty-level incomes are sufficient to provide all a family needs to maintain good health and, second, from misconceptions about expenditure patterns on non-essential goods, such as alcohol or video recorders. With the exception of expenditure on tobacco, low-income families spend significantly smaller proportions of their income on non-essential goods than higher-income families. Many low-income families may have video recorders, but video-recorder repayments or hire charges are often the only weekly expenditure on leisure goods/activities in the household.

Women's accounts of family poverty suggest that financial arrangements within the home influence budgeting patterns and the distribution of health resources within the family. In many families day-to-day management of the household budget tends to be women's responsibility. The evidence suggests that, when women are able to implement their own spending priorities, they can modify the effects of poverty on family members through juggling the budget each week. When male partners control family spending priorities, the worst effects of family poverty are less likely to be contained. Women appear to mitigate the effect of poverty on other family members by cutting down on their own consumption and expenditure. In lone-mother families the distinction between control and management of money is dissolved. Lone mothers' accounts of living on a low income suggest that, although they have lower incomes than two-parent families, they may find it easier to contain the worst aspects of family poverty through careful management of the household budget and by cutting their personal consumption and expenditure.

To conclude, the evidence indicates that the expenditure patterns and lifestyles of low-income families cannot be explained in terms of budgeting skills, health attitudes or knowledge levels. Household spending on health resources, such as food, heating, clothing, transport, safety equipment and social activities, appears to be closely associated with the level of income which is available to families. To understand the relationship between poverty and family health, it is necessary to understand the role that income plays in family life.

THE ROLE OF INCOME IN FAMILY HEALTH

Family health is dependent on both economic and human resources.[1] Household income is the medium through which many economic resources reach the family. It is also a resource that influences the conditions under which human resources, usually women, work for family health. A family's access to many health resources is heavily dependent on income levels. Income levels influence both the social and economic circumstances in which people live and their health behaviour. Access to good housing, healthy food, a safe home environment and to health and social facilities all depend, to a large extent, on how much money is available to the household and how it is distributed within it. Household-income levels therefore have a direct influence on an individual's level of exposure to anti-health forces: on exposure to infections and environmental hazards, and on the body's capacity to resist and recover from infections and illness. Household-income levels also determine an individual's degree of domestic comfort and access to social-support networks. Both of these factors make an important contribution to mental and social well-being.

Caring for children, particularly if they have disabilities or are sick, creates the need for extra resources. The evidence we examined suggests those with the highest health-resource needs are least likely to have an income level that is compatible with good health. High unemployment rates and low-paid work, particularly among women and Black and minority ethnic groups means that many families are totally or partially dependent on social-security benefits for their income. Yet, social-security rates are set too low to meet the health and material needs of families with young children. Whilst some social-security benefits have risen in value in real terms over the last decade, they have failed to keep pace with average earnings.

Throughout this book we have seen numerous examples of how low household income prevents families from having access to vital health resources and carrying out health behaviours that are generally considered to be important for good health. Chapters 2 to 6 explored how various dimensions of poverty affect the health of those who experience it. Studies of food poverty indicate how many low-income families cannot afford the foods that are considered important for health. Healthy foods are not only more expensive than less healthy foods, they are also less readily available to families who depend on local shopping facilities. Women appear to bear the brunt of food poverty. By cutting back on their food, they are able reduce the effects of food poverty on other family members. For Black and minority ethnic families, the problems of food poverty are made more difficult because many traditional foods are not readily available. Travelling to buy traditional foods adds to the cost of foods that are already likely to be more expensive due to import costs. The evidence made it clear that many illnesses and conditions that are more common among low-income groups than higher-income groups can be explained in terms of food poverty.

Lack of money for food is not an isolated example of the way poverty restricts access to vital health resources. Low-income families frequently limit the use of heating as a way of making money available for other resources, such as food and clothing. Families with poverty-level incomes cannot afford family outings, or many of the goods that make life more bearable. The extra costs associated with bringing up children are particularly hard to meet. Low-income families find it difficult to purchase safety equipment, such as fire-guards and stair-gates, or buy good-quality household and childcare equipment that will last and measure up to current safety standards.

Many low-income families have housing conditions that are incompatible with good health. We saw that poor housing conditions are experienced disproportionately by low-income families. Low-income families are less likely than other groups to own their homes and more likely to live in damp, overcrowded and poorly constructed properties that are in a state of disrepair. Unhealthy conditions within the home are compounded by unhealthy external environments and geographical locations. As a consequence, low-income families are likely to be exposed to high levels of environmental pollution and environmental dangers, such as the absence of safe play areas, a high volume of traffic, poor street lighting and inadequate measures to protect personal safety. Families in poverty also appear to live in geographical areas which have poor community resources, such as childcare, health-care, education and leisure facilities. In many cases, the facilities themselves are not only less readily available but also often poorly resourced and offer an inferior service.

Lack of choice about housing location and housing design often means that families with young children are housed away from friends and family members. The data suggests that neighbourhoods may not always be able to compensate for this through community social-support structures. It has been demonstrated that high levels of social integration and good social-support networks are important for good mental health. Parenthood and poverty are two experiences that are known to be associated with high levels of stress and depression. Low income is a source of stress and prevents its resolution. Families in poverty are likely to experience more stressful life-events than families with higher-income levels. Poverty brings with it the worry and stress of not having enough money to provide for family health, of not being able to participate in social events in the way that others do, of bills and debts, and the stress associated with poor housing conditions and living in an unsafe environment. For some families, poverty also brings with it a sense of social loss – the loss of loved ones who have suffered the health costs of poverty, and the material losses that low income may bring. Black and minority ethnic families suffer the stress of poverty and more. The accounts of Black and minority ethnic families illustrated how the daily experience of personal and institutional racism compounds the stress of low-income living.

Social-support networks are not only important for mental well-being, they are also a source of help for families. Family, friends and neighbours are important sources of help on a daily basis and in times of crises. Mutual exchanges of material and social help appear to protect families from the worst elements of poverty. However, it appears that those who experience the lowest incomes live in areas where the least help is available.

The way poverty shapes family health care has been a recurrent theme throughout the book. Income levels influence the conditions under which families care for their health. Poverty influences how parents care for their chldren's health, and how they care for their own health. A range of studies remind us that family health behaviours and practices do not occur in a social vacuum. They are influenced by the social and economic circumstances of people's lives. Throughout this book, parents' own accounts of their experiences of poverty have illustrated how health-related behaviour is modified and constrained by two issues: control and compromise.

Parents' own descriptions of caring provided us with graphic accounts of how low income makes it difficult to exercise control over family health. Poverty means that families have very little control relative to other groups over where they live, or how they live. Parents' descriptions of the way they cope with poverty remind us that low-income parents are not passive in the face of difficulty. Whilst poverty reduces the amount of power and control parents have over family health care, parents appear to go to great lengths to take control over those parts of their lives which they can control. Low-income parents appear to cope with the lack of control that poverty imposes by making compromises. Compromising health needs and health activities is not unique to low-income families. Compromise is an inherent part of family life. However, for families on low income, compromises appear to be the greatest and have the most profound effects on family health.

Three main types of compromises can be discerned from parents' accounts of family health care. First, caring for family health in poverty means compromising one health activity in favour of another. Second, caring for family health in poverty means compromising the health needs of parents in favour of the health needs of children. By cutting back on personal consumption parents reconcile the necessity to minimize the effects of low income and maximize the health of their children. Third, caring for family health in poverty often means compromising one family member's health needs for the needs of other family members. Women's smoking behaviour falls into this category of compromise. One of the reasons why women say they continue to smoke, even though it has costs for the family budget and their personal health, is because it allows them to cope with the demands of caring for family health in poverty. By compromising their own health, they promote the health of others.

Our knowledge about the links between poverty and health is incomplete. However, we have enough evidence to suggest that poverty has a major impact on health. The poor health of families in poverty cannot be explained in terms of their failure to adopt desirable attitudes to health. The health effects of poverty stem from the way low income and poor access to health resources influence the social and economic environment in which families live, and the climate within which they care for families within the home.

Poverty affects health in a complex way. This book identified a framework within which the links between poverty and health could be analysed. Whilst this framework is somewhat artificial, separating out processes that, in reality, are intertwined, the exercise is useful for two main reasons. First, it gives some indication of the key processes by which poverty shapes the health status of individuals and families. Second, it indicates how poverty affects every aspect of health: physical, psychological and behavioural. The relationship between poverty and health cannot be understood by analyses that rest on behavioural explanations alone, or on those concentrating solely on material factors. Poverty influences both the conditions in which families live and the climate in which they care.

IMPLICATIONS FOR POLICY AND PRACTICE

As we move into the 1990s, health and welfare workers often have few expectations for radical change: horizons are narrow and optimism limited. However, it is still important to maintain a sense of what policies are needed – perhaps even more important when opportunities for doing more than 'holding the line' are limited. The scale of poverty in Britain cannot be ignored, nor is it likely to diminish significantly in the near future. Tackling poverty is central to any policy initiatives that aim not only to increase family well-being, but also to promote social justice and reduce inequalities in health. The causes of poverty are varied and complex, and no single strategy alone is likely to solve the problems of poverty and poor health. The evidence suggests that poverty needs to be tackled on two main, but inter-related fronts – on the social-policy front and on the health- and welfare-practice front.

SOCIAL POLICY INTO THE 1990s
The evidence we have reviewed points to some clear directions for social policy. Tackling poverty and its associated health and social problems will require a range of policy initiatives across the field of social policy. The picture of family poverty that has emerged suggests that two elements are essential in formulating policy related to poverty:

Policies need to provide families and individuals in and out of employment with a level of income and material resources that is compatible with good health.

Policies need to tackle structures that lock certain groups – women, Black and minority ethnic groups, people with disabilities, and people who work in less secure and less valued sectors of the labour market – into poverty and disadvantage over a lifetime.

The remainder of this sub-section will concentrate on some of the main policy changes that are needed to improve the health and welfare of Britain's families.

Improving employment and wage policies form a central part of any strategy that aims to decrease poverty. Income through employment is the major source of household income for families with children. Unemployment and low pay remain the major causes of poverty for families in Britain.

Reducing poverty, therefore, means reducing unemployment by improving and equalizing access to jobs, particularly well-paid and secure jobs. The introduction of a minimum wage is a key way of ensuring that all families with working adults have incomes above the poverty line. Tackling poverty through unemployment also means improving access to well-paid and secure jobs for Black and minority ethnic people, through training schemes and recruitment policies that remove the racial barriers that force many Black and minority ethnic workers into the worst jobs, with the lowest pay and least security.

Tackling women's poverty through employment and wage policies is central to any anti-poverty strategy. Poverty levels are higher among women than men, and women bear the brunt of poverty in the home. Wage policies need to ensure decent wages for women, and wages that are equal to men's. Women also need employment policies that promote access to better-paid and higher-status jobs and, once they have them, women need policies that enable them to keep them. This will involve improving women's access to employment after childbirth and periods of unpaid caring away from work through a number of measures. Improved employment rights would allow more women to take paid maternity leave and return to the same job if they wish. Improved, cheaper and more readily available childcare facilities are an essential prerequisite if women are to take up employment: the quality, range, costs and availability of childcare services remain a key issue in women's poverty. Changes in the provision of education and training for women will contribute to improving women's position in the employment market. Tackling women's poverty is also dependent on policies that encourage male partners to take on a greater share of caring within the home. More flexible working hours would allow both parents to combine paid work with unpaid caring responsibilities. Extended parental leave, available to either parent on the birth of a child, and at times when children are ill, would allow fathers to participate more fully in family health care, and both parents to combine the demands of paid work with those of unpaid work in the home with greater ease.

Improving income maintenance through the social-security system is a crucial mechanism through which household incomes can be increased. The inadequacy of the income-maintenance system has been a recurrent theme throughout this book. It was clear that income-support premiums need to be raised, particularly for children and expectant mothers. The evidence also suggests that the income-support system needs to recognize that income requirements alter with changing personal and family circumstances. Unlike the supplementary-benefit system, the income-support system fails to provide additional help when families' circumstances change or additional costs are incurred. The social fund fails to plug the gap which was left when single payments under the supplementary-benefit system were abolished. The need to reverse the trend away from means-tested benefits to universal benefits is also clear. Research has shown that universal benefits, such as child benefit, are crucial benefits to families and have high take-up rates. Many means-tested benefits, like family credit, have low rates of take up and often fail to meet the needs of those with the greatest needs. The need to improve access to and take up of benefits is clear. Ensuring that people get the benefits they are entitled to at least improves the standard of living for some families, even if it cannot lift them out of poverty. The social-security system is complicated both to administer and for families to approach. Improved access to social-security benefits is particularly crucial to raising the living standards of Black and minority ethnic families. Many Black and minority ethnic families experience considerable difficulties obtaining social-security benefits.

Families need policies that recognize the additional costs that children bring and help them to meet these costs. Child benefit, the only universally available additional concession to parents, has been shown to be a crucial benefit, particularly to mothers. The future of child benefit, as a universal benefit, is uncertain. What is certain is that it is now worth less, in real terms, than in 1979. Improving child benefit is an important way of helping families to meet the additional costs of children. Free school meals to children from low-income families are also an important way of ensuring that children at least get one meal a day. The numbers of children who are eligible for free school meals has fallen over the past two decades. Today only children from families who are in receipt of income support are eligible. Other children from low-income families, for example, from homes in receipt of family credit, or those with incomes who are just above the threshold for family credit, are excluded.

Families with people with disabilities need income maintenance policies that fully recognize the costs of caring. The Disability Alliance suggests that a comprehensive disability-income scheme is needed to prevent poverty among families with people with disabilities and bring their living standards up to those of comparable other families. They suggest that there should be three elements to this scheme. First, a disablement allowance, which would vary according to a person's disability, should be paid to all people with long-term disabilities, regardless of age or employment status. Second, a disablement pension should be paid as an income-maintenance benefit to all people with disabilities who are incapable of work, regardless of whether they have paid enough national insurance contributions or not. Third, a carer's pension should be paid to carers of working age who are prevented from working because they care for an adult or child with a disability.

Families need housing policies that provide them with housing conditions that are conducive to good health. Housing policies need to address the shortage of homes for families through house-building programmes. A relaxation of public-sector borrowing controls would allow local authorities to spend more on house-building and renovation programmes themselves and co-operate with the private sector and housing associations to provide family homes. New and renovated properties need to be built according to standards and regulations that work towards the elimination of damp, overcrowding and unsafe conditions, excessive heat loss and noise pollution. Town-planning policies need to ensure that family homes are built in locations that improve personal safety, have plentiful play areas for children, low levels of traffic and environmental pollution and easy access to health, education, leisure and shopping facilities. Housing inequalities for Black and minority ethnic families, over and above those of white families, compound problems of poverty. Eradicating or reducing the effects of poverty for Black and minority ethnic families demands that local housing authorities develop housing policies that remove racial discrimination in housing through allocation and exchange procedures. Until healthy family homes become a reality for families in poverty, resources that help families cope and avoid the worst effects of adverse conditions are necessary. Improved local childcare facilities are needed for children of parents who are not in paid employment, in order to allow them to spend time away from the health hazards of damp, cold, overcrowded and poorly designed homes, and to offer parents a break from the stress of caring for young children in unhealthy housing.

Families in poverty need health policies that are responsive to their health needs. Poor families need better access to local preventive and curative health services. Chapter 6 indicated that those with the most health needs often have the poorest access to health services, and receive poor-quality services in comparison to other groups. Health policies at national and local level need to provide the opportunity for families to receive services that are responsive to the needs of communities. Whilst many health authorities have begun to collect data on how social and economic factors influence the health of local communities, there is still a long way to go before these data are incorporated into routine planning. Health policy makers need to develop better strategies for evaluating the effect that services have on the health of local communities. Health indicators need to form the basis for this evaluation. The present trend towards the development of service-performance indicators is unlikely to provide information on the impact that policies have had on the health and welfare of the community.

Health-promotion policies exert a strong influence on the health and welfare of families. The evidence reviewed here suggests that many health-promotion policies fail to recognize the way poverty influences family health and family health-care activities. Policy-makers have an obligation to re-examine many of the assumptions that underlie current health-promotion programmes. In particular, they need to question the assumption that poor families can choose healthy lifestyles in the face of poverty. This assumption forms the basis of many health-promotion policies today. The recognition that poverty has an important bearing on family health is not only likely to lead to policies that are responsive to the needs of families, but to health promotion policies that seek to challenge the structural causes of family poverty and poor family health.

Tackling family poverty, in the final analysis, demands policies that seek to tackle social-class inequalities, sexism and racism in Britain. Social class, gender and 'race' divisions shape the way health resources are distributed between and within groups. Policies for the 1990s should recognize that improving family health rests on strategies which at the very least begin to reduce poverty and social inequalities.

HEALTH AND WELFARE WORK: WHAT DIRECTION NOW?

It is important to acknowledge that, without social-policy changes, health and welfare work cannot alone tackle the health and social costs of family poverty. However, it is the shape of health and welfare practice itself that has an important influence on families in poverty. There is a two-way relationship between health and welfare work on the one hand and family poverty on the other. First, family poverty and its consequences for family health create a major reason why families become users of health and welfare services. Poor families are heavy users of health and welfare services, and substantial proportions of health and welfare resources are directly and indirectly absorbed by them. Second, the nature of health and welfare interventions has an influence on how families experience poverty and poor health problems. When health and welfare workers provide services that are flexible and responsive to the needs of families in poverty, they can help families cope with and avoid the worst effects of poverty. At its best, health and welfare work can provide a challenge to policy-makers to develop strategies that reduce poverty. At its worst, it serves to compound the effect of poverty on family life and family health.

Although health and welfare workers play a crucial role in the lives of many families, it is important to recognize that there is no single solution that can be adopted by fieldworkers and used in their work. The social events and trends of the 1980s and early 1990s mean that, although agencies face some common issues relating to poverty, they also face problems that are unique to their own agencies and to the communities they serve. First, poverty is not experienced uniformly by neighbourhoods or by social groups within neighbourhoods. Second, agencies do not necessarily share ideologies, remits for intervention or similar levels of resources. Third, health and welfare services have been, and continue to be, extensively restructured. Reforms have had different consequences for individual agencies and their work. Perhaps the most valuable lesson we can learn from the research on poverty and family health is that no blueprint can be applied uniformly across communities or health and welfare agencies. The details of strategies and solutions need to be worked out with individual communities, and within and across agencies. Although instant answers are not available, research on poverty and health offers us some invaluable insights into the direction that health and welfare needs to take if it is to develop more sensitive and appropriate strategies for working with families in poverty. Three key points emerge from the research and literature reviewed in this book.

First, any health and welfare strategy that aims to improve family health and the ability of families to meet their own needs should have family poverty as its central concern. Family poverty needs to be a central item on the agenda of health and welfare work. Studies indicate that health and welfare work often fails to identify family poverty as its prime concern. Practice has tended to respond at the margins of family poverty and health problems. Interventions are often reactive, responding to the consequences of family poverty rather than to the roots of the problems. Studies of poverty-awareness among health and welfare workers suggest that, for family poverty to become a central issue for practice, individual workers and agencies need to increase their levels of poverty awareness.[2] Although health and welfare workers may recognize that poverty is an extensive social problem, they do not necessarily see what they do as related to poverty. Much health and welfare work is not based on either an awareness of poverty as an issue or on a sound knowledge base concerning the effect of poverty on family life and family health.

There is evidence to suggest that financial and material problems tend to be disguised or redefined as issues of personal or emotional inadequacy[3] – as the failure of families to cope with their living conditions, as personal health problems that stem from undesirable attitudes to health and child-care, as skills and knowledge deficits and as irresponsible personal behaviour. Those workers who do recognize the relationship between the structural nature of poverty and their work with families often feel power-less and unable to make an impact on poverty and poor health. The recognition that poverty has structural rather than personal causes under-standably raises questions in workers' minds about their ability to have any real influence on the problems that poor families face. Whilst it is important to recognize that health and welfare work is likely to have little impact on the structural causes of poverty, nevertheless health and welfare work has an important bearing on family health and family poverty. It is essential therefore that this impact is positive.

Increasing levels of poverty awareness among workers are the first, and perhaps most difficult, step to take along the road towards making family poverty of central concern in health and welfare work. Health and welfare work needs to evaluate the extent to which practice is influenced by attitudes to poverty and poor clients at two levels – at the individual level and the organizational level. Individual workers and organizations need to assess and evaluate how personal and organizational attitudes and values inhibit and distort the focus of their work. For many people, this will be a painful experience, and one that cannot be completed without encouragement and support from colleagues and managers. The studies reviewed in this book remind us that an examination of personal and organizational attitudes to poverty and poor families cannot be successfully completed without an examination of how attitudes to 'race' and gender affect health and welfare work.

Many attitudes to family poverty and the health needs of poor families are embodied in health and welfare strategies and methods of intervention. Making poverty a central issue in health and welfare work requires that workers and organizations examine whether strategies and methods of intervention should be modified. Individuals and teams of workers need to ask whether their strategies and methods reflect an awareness of both the structural nature of poverty and the impact of poverty on family life and family health. Many agencies will have to become better informed about the processes that create and maintain family poverty locally and nationally. Workers will find it useful to build up poverty profiles that document and analyse the extent of poverty in local areas and its social and health costs to families. The material reviewed in this book reminds us that both facts and figures and family accounts of poverty and poor health provide us with a valuable information base on which to draw when making decisions about work with families. For some teams of workers this will involve extending information systems to collect poverty data, whilst others will need to build new systems to collect appropriate information on poverty. Titterton[4] suggests that evaluation should be placed at the centre of this renewed concern for family poverty. He identifies the requirement for two types of evaluative activity: the evaluation of the distribution of poverty among those who receive interventions, and the evaluation of outcomes of specific types of intervention. Little progress has been made in either of these areas, yet only with this new knowledge will teams of workers be able to consider how they should be responding at the neighbourhood, local and national level, as individuals and organizations, to poverty and health issues.

A second key point that emerges from the literature is that inter-agency collaboration should be a fundamental aspect of any strategy that aims to tackle the health and welfare concerns of poor families. Health and welfare work needs to respond in a way that recognizes that financial, health and social problems are inseparable and that they stem from the same set of social and economic factors. Families tell us that they do not experience these problems as separate problems. Yet health and welfare work has a tendency to separate out financial, health and social problems and treat them as discrete entities. Individual agencies tend to focus on separate sets of presenting problems. As a result, fieldwork responses to family poverty and poor health are often fragmented. The value of inter-agency work lies in its ability to move fieldwork practice away from trying to find individual solutions to problems that are rooted in social and economic factors.

The case for greater collaboration and more integrative methods of

intervention between health and welfare agencies and between the statutory and the voluntary sector has been advocated for several decades. Since
the 1970s, there has been a growth of interest in the development of
neighbourhood and community-orientated initiatives in both the statutory
and voluntary sectors. The majority of health and social-service departments now work in neighbourhood teams. However, the fact that many
local health authorities, social-service departments and education departments do not have boundaries that are coterminous prevents agencies from
working together effectively. Whilst there has been a growth in inter-agency
collaboration, it typically remains on the margins of mainstream health and
welfare work. The challenge to health and welfare agencies in the 1990s is to
move towards building networks between agencies. Inter-agency collaboration needs to be accepted both as a central strategy and as a method in
health and welfare work. This calls for networks to be built at both the
organizational level and the level of fieldwork practice. Many inter-agency
initiatives have failed simply because collaboration at fieldwork level has
not had the support of managers. Workers will need to seek ways of
increasing their knowledge of what other agencies do, and how they work
with families. This will mean checking out whether the assumptions we
hold about other agencies are correct and being prepared to work out a
common understanding of which skills are unique to each agency and
which are common to all.

As we have seen in earlier chapters of this book, parents' accounts of
parenting in poverty suggest several types of provision are key resources to
families in poverty. First, families value facilities and services that help
them to mitigate and cope with the material effects and stress of breadline
living. Food co-operatives, cheap community transport, shopping schemes,
community eating facilities, more childcare provision, local welfare-rights
advice services and after-school schemes for school-age children are all
initiatives that have been shown to be important resources to families in
poverty. Parents appear to welcome the opportunity to meet together in
groups to learn from each other and to provide and receive social support.
The need for good social-support networks has been a recurrent theme
throughout this book. The evidence suggests that health and welfare
workers urgently need to develop and extend their role in the area of
stimulating and maintaining neighbourhood support networks. Where
health and welfare resources are scarce, or workers lack confidence to set up
and run self-help and social-support groups, co-working across agencies can
be a mechanism by which resources are pooled, costs are shared and skills
exchanged. Statutory agencies have many valuable lessons to learn from
voluntary agencies who have taken the lead in demonstrating the scope for
preventive work with families, based on locally organized and integrated
services such as family clubs, family centres, parent and toddler groups and
women's groups.[5]

The third key point that emerges from this exploration of the research is that parents want the opportunity to care for family health in partnership with health and welfare workers. Working in partnership with parents means valuing the contribution that individual families make to family health care. Families are not passive recipients of health care, they are the main providers of care for the family. Partnership means acknowledging that families recognize their responsibility for health and exercise it on a daily basis. Professionals only make a small input into the totality of family health care. When professionals talk of 'giving families back the responsibility for health and welfare' and getting them 'to take more responsibility for health', they are failing to acknowledge and understand how family health care is constructed.

Working in partnership also means seeing diversity as a strength.[6] The contradictions and compromises that are inherent parts of family life mean that workers need to acknowledge that there is no right way of doing things. There are no 'ideal' family structures, methods of child-rearing or health care. Families need to work out their own solutions. Families ask for services which give them the information on which they can base decisions and the support to carry out what they decide. Partnership relationships with families demand that health and welfare workers question many of the assumptions they have about family life and family care. They mean listening to families and accepting what they themselves identify as their needs and concerns, rather than the imposition of professional agendas. Listening to what families say means building mechanisms whereby families can be listened to at all levels, from the level of individual contact with workers to participation in the planning of services. Clearly working in partnership raises contradictions for workers who have to exercise statutory responsibilities, for example, social workers working in the area of child protection. The political climate in which statutory responsibilities are currently exercised in childcare work has forced workers to rely on legislative, rather than voluntary, arrangements.

Families appear to appreciate individual contact when health and welfare workers value the family health-care work they do. Families want health and welfare workers to acknowledge the constraints under which they carry out this work, particularly the compromises and contradictions that mothers face in their unpaid health work. The valuable insights that studies on health and poverty bring also help health and welfare workers to formulate advice for families that is achievable within the limits of low income. As we saw in chapter 3, 'throw away the chip pan' type advice is more likely to compound poverty and health problems than to alleviate them. Families want information on social-security benefits and on using the social-security system. Women want help to gain access to childcare facilities and information about other forms of social support in the community.

Parents underline the importance of easy access to services, particularly child health services. Parents often find services difficult to use because they are in the wrong location, open at inconvenient times, involve long waiting times or are not welcoming. Moreover, many buildings which families visit to receive services, such as housing offices, social-service offices, social-security offices and health centres, are not designed with parents with young children in mind. Parents also ask for services that provide high levels of expertise.

For many workers, developing health and welfare strategies and methods of intervention which are sensitive to the needs of families in poverty and encompass partnership styles of work may prove to be a difficult experience. Facing one's own attitudes to poverty and family work and questioning the styles of work that are familiar and comfortable cannot be undertaken without encouragement and support. Intra-agency and inter-agency approaches can enable neighbourhood workers and managers to go through this process together. They allow workers to move forward in a common direction and towards a common goal, whilst at the same time providing and receiving support from fellow workers. The trend towards the decentralization of learning and training provides an ideal opportunity to make family poverty a central part of health and welfare work. Taking training and staff development to neighbourhood teams will enable workers to develop strategies that reflect the diversity of needs within and between neighbourhoods and that recognize the local constraints that they face.

Poverty and its associated effects on family health remain an important issue for health and welfare policy and practice as we move through the 1990s. There are few signs that the climate in which family health care takes place will undergo any significant changes for the better in the near future. Health and welfare workers will continue to provide a backbone of support for low-income families in the 1990s, but in the face of new challenges and new constraints. Although we can have few expectations of radical change, it is important that we maintain a sense of optimism. Health and welfare workers provide essential support services to families on low income, and there remains the opportunity to work towards the development of more flexible and responsive services for families.

REFERENCES

1 Graham, H. (1984). *Women, Health and the Family*. Brighton, Wheatsheaf.
2 Becker, S. (1988). 'Poverty awareness', in Becker, S., MacPherson, S. (eds) *Public Issues, Private Pain*. London, Social Services Insight.
3 Jordan, B. (1988). 'Poverty, social work and the state', in Becker, S. and MacPherson, S. (eds) (1988). op. cit.
4 Titterton, M. (1988). 'Evaluating social work services for the poor', in Becker, S. and MacPherson, S. (eds) (1988). op. cit.
5 Holman, B. (1988). *Putting Families First: Prevention and Childcare*. London, Macmillan.
6 Brown, D. (1990). 'Introduction: values and purposes of family education', *Journal of Community Education*, vol. 8, 4.

INDEX